Acute Leukemia

Difficult, Controversial, Automated Analysis

Acute Leukemia
Difficult, Controversial, Automated Analysis

HAROLD R. SCHUMACHER, MD

Professor of Pathology
University of Cincinnati Medical Center
Medical Director, Hematology Service
Alliance Laboratory Services
Director, Hematopathology
Fellowship Program
Cincinnati, Ohio

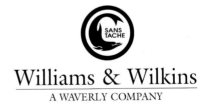

Williams & Wilkins
A WAVERLY COMPANY

BALTIMORE • PHILADELPHIA • LONDON • PARIS • BANGKOK
BUENOS AIRES • HONG KONG • MUNICH • SYDNEY • TOKYO • WROCLAW

Editor: David Charles Retford
Managing Editors: Lynn Johnston & Jennifer Eckhoff
Marketing Manager: Daniell Griffin
Production Coordinator: Marette D. Magargle-Smith
Project Editor: Jennifer D. Weir
Designer: Dan Pfisterer
Cover Designer: Dan Pfisterer
Typesetter: Maryland Composition Inc.
Printer & Binder: Transcontinental Printing Inc.

Copyright © 1998 Williams & Wilkins
351 West Camden Street
Baltimore, Maryland 21201-2436 USA
Rose Tree Corporate Center
1400 North Providence Road
Building II, Suite 5025
Media, Pennsylvania 19063-2043 USA

Printed in Canada

Library of Congress Cataloging-in-Publication Data
Schumacher, Harold R. (Harold Robert)
    Acute Leukemia: difficult, controversial, automated analysis /
Harold R. Schumacher.—1st ed.
      p. cm.
    Includes index.
    ISBN 0-683-30505-0
    1. Leukemia—Cytodiagnosis 2. Leukemia—Immunodiagnosis.
  3. Leukemia—Cytodiagnosis—Automation.
    RC643.S375 1997
    616.99´419075—dc21   97-34124

To purchase additional copies of this book, call our customer service department at **(800) 638-0672** or fax orders to **(800) 447-8438.** For other book services, including chapter reprints and large quantity sales, ask for the Special Sales department.
Canadian customers should call **(800) 665-1148**, or fax **(800) 665-0103.** For all other calls originating outside of the United States, please call **(410) 528-4223** or fax us at **(410) 528-8550.**

Visit Williams & Wilkins on the Internet: **http://www.wwilkins.com** or contact our customer service department at **custserv@wwilkins.com.** Williams & Wilkins customer service representatives are available from 8:30 am to 6:00 pm, EST, Monday through Friday, for telephone access.

97 98 99 00 01
1 2 3 4 5 6 7 8 9 10

To my children, with all my love:
Robert, Gail, Steven, Mary, Karen

To those who understand me
To those who don't
To those who never thought about it

Foreword

This monograph is the expert compilation of Dr. Harold R. Schumacher's vast experience with the acute leukemias, and is a timely and fitting update to his earlier book entitled "Acute Leukemia: Approach to Diagnosis," published by Igaku-Shoin in 1990.

During the past 170 years, since the first description of leukemia by Velpeau in 1827, a vast body of knowledge about the acute leukemias has accrued, with concurrent refinements in diagnostic technique and therapy.

Following the recommendations of the FAB group in 1976, the acute leukemias have been classified into definable groups. Similarly, the chronic leukemias and myelodysplastic syndromes have been organized into meaningful classifications.

In recent years, the scope of hematopathology has been broadened, with ever widening expectations to specifically identify leukemic subtypes. Candidates pursuing certification in Hematology, Oncology, Pathology, and Hematopathology are now challenged to recognize specific entities and newer therapeutic modalities that have made the expectation of cure a reality in some subtypes.

The structure and composition of the marrow fortunately lends itself to cytologic, histologic, and esoteric testing, and in recent years increasing numbers of centers are conserving resources and modifying organizational detail to centralize diagnostic hematopathology services. During the years following my fellowship with Dr. Schumacher, I have come to firmly believe in his teaching that the clinical profile, CBC, peripheral smear, aspirate, core biopsy, iron stain, touch preps, cytochemistry, immunohistochemistry, immunophenotype, ultrastructure, and analysis of cytokines should be considered as independent resources, each capable of providing valuable diagnostic information.

All nine chapters of this monograph are invaluable to the diagnostician and the researcher. Recent advances beyond the FAB group's recommendations, such as the subclassification of erythroleukemia (AML-M6), the biphenotypic leukemias, and in the areas of cytogenetics, molecular genetics, cytokines, and immunophenotyping make this a well-tabulated and referenced repository of current knowledge. Additionally, a valuable and totally new approach describing the evaluation of the acute leukemias by automated Abbott Cell-Dyn Systems is outlined while representative case studies bring balance to this work. Dr. Schumacher's monograph will be a welcome addition to my library and is recommended to all interested in this challenging subject.

James D. Cotelingam, MD
Head, Hematopathology and Professor of Pathology
Director, Clinical Laboratories
Louisiana State University Medical Center
Shreveport, Louisiana   71130

Preface

The primary objective of this book is to provide updated additional basic and practical knowledge on the acute leukemias beyond the French-American-British (FAB) classification. Although morphology and cytochemistry continue to be the mainstays of the diagnosis of acute leukemia, new developments in immunophenotyping, cytogenetics, molecular biology, and in vitro assays have dramatically improved our understanding of this disease and enabled the identification of new entities with distinct clinicobiologic features. In addition, this work gives us a glimpse of the now and future in automated hematologic instrumentation. Again, the multifaceted unified approach is emphasized in order to arrive at a correct diagnosis. The book is readable and succinct; however, the pertinent information has been retained.

New chapters on morphology, cytochemistry, immunophenotyping, cytogenetics, molecular genetics, cytokines, and automated hematologic instrumentation provide the prerequisite knowledge to diagnose those acute leukemias beyond the FAB classification. The chapter on morphology addresses unique morphological features of these unusual leukemias. The chapter on cytochemistry is brief, and relates to the new entities. Transmission electron microscopy was included in appropriate areas throughout the book. The chapter on immunophenotyping emphasizes the impact of this burgeoning field on the understanding and definition of these new unique leukemias. Equally, cytogenetics has revealed some unusual associations that are clinically relevant for diagnosis, for example, t(15;17)(q22;q12); t(1;19)(q23; p13). Recently, interphase cytogenetics has served to broaden the scope and utility of cytogenetic analysis beyond the limits of conventional metaphase-based technology. Also, the book discusses the impact of molecular genetics and cytokines on the acute leukemias in general. Finally, a chapter on automated hematology analyzers with emphasis on the Abbott Cell-Dyn instrument Systems with their emerging technology completes the chapters in the first section.

The second portion of the book provides practical information in the form of cases analyzed by automated hematology analyzers (Abbott Cell-Dyn 3500 and 4000 systems). Such analysis provides initial screening data that, in some cases, may direct the hematologist/hematopathologist/pathologist toward the correct classification. The instrument has the capability of detecting small numbers of blast cells and characterizing them according to size, shape, and granularity. Finally, we have included some bone marrow aspirate patterns in the last portion of the book. We have evaluated over 100 samples and have gained new insights into cellular analysis of the acute leukemias. This instrument tickles our imagination because, not too far in the future, such instruments will be capable of morphologic and immunophenotypic analysis on peripheral blood, bone marrow aspirates, lymph nodes, lymphocytic infiltrates, and body fluids. Therefore, it behooves all of us to become aware and knowledgeable of such instrumentation as technology marches into the future. Indeed, if a computer can beat the world champion grand master in chess, certainly automated hematology analyzers of the future should be able to diagnose hematologic diseases as well as hematologists/ hematopathologists.

The author sincerely hopes that this book will be an easy source of learning about unique, acute leukemias and new instrumentation as we approach the next century and new millennium. The book should be of great interest to those who must deal with the diagnosis and treatment of the acute leukemias.

Acknowledgments

The author is most indebted to a number of people who, through their efforts, support, and cooperation, made this book possible.

A very special thanks to my secretary Pat Hathaway who typed and edited the entire manuscript. She also maintained accurate files, sent and received permission letters, and communicated with the editor and his staff.

The author owes a special gratitude to Dr. Fermina Mazzella, fellow in hematopathology, who read and edited the entire manuscript, obtained articles and reviews from the library, and ran many of the peripheral blood and bone marrows through the automated hematology analyzers (Cell-Dyn 3500, 4000). Without her tenacity of purpose, curiosity, and dedication, this book would not have been possible. Also, my thanks to Dr. Luke Wibowo, former fellow, who helped with the early stages of the book. Additionally, the author is indebted to another former fellow, Dr. Atef Shrit, who provided case material for the book.

Thanks to Dr. Ann Murray, a pathology resident who was very helpful in supplying articles and reviews on the unusual and controversial acute leukemias from the University of Cincinnati Medical Center Library.

Outstanding photographic support was provided by Jay Card, who developed, duplicated, and photographed most of the material within the book.

Additional gratitude is extended to technologists Jody Reisinger, Brenda Paulson, and Kim Walker for their expert technical assistance and advice. They were responsible for processing many of the peripheral bloods and bone marrow specimens that were illustrated in the book. In addition, they prepared many of the cytochemical stains. Also, my thanks to Joyce Collier who prepared the histological sections and immunohistochemical stains.

Further, special recognition should be given to Lois Roberts for her technical expertise of the automated instrumentation. In addition, she supplied much of the hematological data and scattergrams in many of the cases.

Excellent medical illustration was furnished by John Klancher and Deb Havelka.

Thanks to Dr. Paul Steele who gave advice on the Molecular Genetics and Cytokines chapters.

The author is indebted to Drs. Ralph Gruppo, Paul Jubinsky, and Cindy DeLaat for supplying clinical information, laboratory data, and slides on pediatric cases.

A special debt of gratitude is extended to Dr. Ruth Blough and her technologists, Lori Reimer, Margie Hayes, and Linda Shepard, who provided the karyotypes, fluorescent in situ hybridization (FISH), and whole chromosome paint illustrations that appear in this book. Also, thanks again to Dr.

Ruth Blough for reviewing the chapter on cytogenetics and offering helpful suggestions.

Finally, the author owes a very special acknowledgment to John Glazier for his technical review.

The author greatly appreciated the support, cooperation, and opportunity to work with the above contributors. Without their help this book would not have been possible.

Abbreviations

ABL	Acute basophilic leukemia
ADC	Analog-to-digital converter
A-EST	Alpha naphthyl acetate esterase
ALIPs	Abnormal localization of immature precursors
ALL	Acute lymphoblastic leukemia
ALL-HMV	Acute lymphoblastic leukemia-hand-mirror variant
AMC	Amoeboid movement configuration
AML	Acute myeloid leukemia
AMLL	Acute mixed lineage leukemia
ANKCL	Aggressive natural killer cell leukemia
AP	Acid phosphatase
Ara-C	Arabinosylcytosine
ATG	Antithymocyte globulin
ATRA	All-transretinoic acid
AUL	Acute undifferentiated leukemia
B-EST	Alpha naphthyl butyrate esterase
BG	Betaglucuronidase
BL	Basophilic leukemia
CAE	Chloroacetate esterase
CALLA	Common acute lymphoblastic leukemia associated antigen
C-EST	Combined esterase
CML	Chronic myelogenous leukemia
CSF	Colony stimulating factor
DCC	Deleted in colorectal carcinoma
DIC	Disseminated intravascular coagulation
DNA	Deoxyribonucleic acid
EL	Eosinophilic leukemia
EM	Electron microscopy
FAB	French-American-British
Fe stain	Iron stain
G-CSF	Granulocyte colony stimulating factor
GM-CSF	Granulocyte macrophage colony stimulating factor
HAML	Hypocellular AML
HeNe	Helium-neon
HES	Hypereosinophilic syndrome
HMC	Hand mirror cells
IRF-1	Interferon regulatory factor
LAP	Leukocyte alkaline phosphatase
LASER	Light amplification by stimulated emission radiation
LGL	Large granular lymphocyte
M.A.P.S.S.	Multi-angle polarized scatter separation
MDR	Multidrug resistance

MDS	Myelodysplastic syndromes
MGP	Methyl green pyronine
MIC	Morphology, Immunology, Cytogenetics
MPEX	Myeloperoxidase
MRD	Minimal residual disease
NASDA	Naphthyl-ASD-acetate
NASDA-F	NASDA with fluoride
N/C ratio	Nuclear-to-cytoplasmic ratio
NEC	Nonerythroid cells
NK	Natural killer
NSE	Nonspecific esterase
NWBC	Non-white blood cell
ORO	Oil red O
PAS	Periodic acid-Schiff
PCNA	Proliferating cell nuclear antigen
PCR	Polymerase chain reaction
Ph^1	Philadelphia chromosome
RAEB-IT	Refractory anemia with excess blasts in transformation
RAR-α	Retinoic acid receptor α
RBC	Red blood cell count
RDW	Red cell distribution width
RNA	Ribonucleic acid
RT-PCR	Reverse transcriptase PCR
SBB	Sudan black B
SEp	Standard error of proportion
TCR	T cell receptor
TdT	Terminal deoxynucleotidyl transferase
TGF	Transforming growth factor
TNF	Tumor necrosis factor
TPO	Thrombopoietin
WBC	White blood cell count
WIC	WBC impedance count
WOC	WBC optical count
WVF	White viable fraction

Contents

Overview

This book supports a statement made by Dr. Sanford Stass at a Society for Hematopathology meeting in *Dallas* in *1990*. At the beginning of the talk he asked the question "What can a leukemic cell do?" After expounding on the complex intricate details of leukemogenesis he answered the question at the end of his talk with "anything it wants." This concept is important to understand since the book deals with unusual, complex cases that fulfill Dr. Stass' assertion.

However complex, morphology and cytochemistry remain the cornerstones for diagnosis, but this is rapidly being eroded by more sophisticated biotechnology. These, like all tests, must be performed with fastidious technological quality and precision, and interpreted by a skilled hematopathologist or hematologist. Utilization of immunophenotyping in diagnosis of leukemia has greatly expanded, largely due to the sophistication and burgeoning expansion of the available monoclonal antibodies. Indeed, immunophenotyping has been added to the cornerstone of morphology and cytochemistry in most laboratories throughout the world. Cytogenetics has slowly fused with molecular genetics and has become increasingly important as we probe the finer nuances of the leukemic cell. Interphase cytogenetics and chromosomal markers have led to improved diagnosis, and have increased our understanding of leukemogenesis. Interestingly, gene rearrangement did not become the court of final appeal. Nevertheless, molecular genetics has impacted greatly on our understanding of leukemia and myelodysplasia. Understanding of the numerous mutations and/or deletions of the RAS family; FMS, MPL genes; and deletions of various tumor suppressor genes, i.e., p53, deleted in colorectal carcinoma (DCC) gene, and interferon regulatory factor (IRF-1) gene, have added new basic knowledge to the complex problem of the leukemic conundrum.

Also, use of the polymerase chain reaction (PCR) has made an impact on minimal residual disease (MRD), albeit with associated interpretive difficulties. Only recently have we begun to investigate and utilize hematopoietic growth factors. They have been employed to some advantage in the treatment of acute leukemias. Ancillary studies may include electron microscopy, which continues to be utilized in the most difficult cases. After having discussed the above complexities of diagnosis, one should never forget that the cardinal sin of misdiagnosis is poor specimen retrieval and substandard slide preparation.

The machine age is upon us! We are rapidly growing more and more reliant upon advancing biotechnology. In this regard, automated hematology analyzers will erode our conventional approach to the diagnosis of acute leukemias and other hematologic disorders. This book reveals incipient insights into the future as our instrumentation becomes ever more complex. Someday in the near future, hematopathologists and hematologists may not even look at slides! Still, whether data comes from the eye and cerebrum or a machine, diagnosis will always involve multifaceted information that will need interpretation and intelligent action by human cognition and intelligence.

CHAPTER 1

Morphology—Difficult and Controversial Acute Leukemias

GENERAL COMMENTS

Although the acute leukemias represent a broad heterogeneous group of malignant disorders, there was a definite need to recognize homogeneous subgroups to improve our understanding of clinical presentation, laboratory features, prognosis, and response to therapy. In 1976, the French-American-British (FAB) Cooperative Group classified the acute leukemias on the basis of peripheral blood and bone marrow evaluation by Romanowsky stains and a battery of cytochemical stains. This classification has been widely accepted; however, the FAB scheme had to be expanded and modified over the years (1982, 1985, 1991) in light of the burgeoning developments in the fields of immunology, cytogenetics, and molecular biology. In this regard, integrated classifications such as that proposed by the Morphology, Immunology, and Cytogenetics (MIC) Cooperative Group have resulted in a reassessment of the leukemic syndromes and provided new diagnostic, prognostic, and therapeutic insights. Further minor refinements were proposed by the National Cancer Institute who proposed that the requisite minimum of blasts for diagnosis of acute leukemia is 30% in blood or bone marrow. Another small variance from the revised FAB proposal, which has virtually no impact on diagnosis or classification, is the form of the differential used in subclassifying acute myeloid leukemia (AML) M1 to AML M5. The FAB committee suggests that subclassification be based on a differential of the nonerythroid myeloid cells. In this book, the subclassification is based on a differential of all marrow cells, including plasma cells and lymphocytes. Finally, the author counts type 1 blasts (no granules) and type 2 blasts (granules up to 21), but not type 3 blasts in the numerical calculation. This book discusses those difficult and controversial acute leukemias that have created problems in diagnosis and classification.

ACUTE UNDIFFERENTIATED LEUKEMIA (AUL)

AUL, unclassifiable by FAB criteria (morphology and cytochemistry), demonstrates signs of immaturity and minimal myeloid and lymphoid differentiation. The impact of biotechnology has eroded the numbers of such cases reported in the literature. Some authors have used the term "stem cell leukemia" as synonymous with AUL, but Yumura-Yagi et al. consider stem cell leukemia to be a subtype of mixed lineage leukemia. Others have used the term "stem cell disorder" to refer to acute myelofibrosis and myelodysplastic syndromes (MDSs). These should not be confused with AUL. The

1

blast cells comprise more than 90% of the marrow cells and are all type I (agranular). The nuclear chromatin is usually fine and two to four variably prominent nuclei may be present. Some blasts may exhibit lymphoid features. Auer rods are not seen. Many cases of AUL have been reclassified on the basis of extensive immunophenotypic analysis and reverse transcriptase polymerase chain reaction (RT-PCR) analysis for myeloperoxidase (MPEX) messenger ribonucleic acid (mRNA).

Undoubtedly, as biotechnology becomes more sophisticated, investigation of genetic abnormalities will more clearly assign lineage to so called undifferentiated leukemia. In this regard, an interstitial deletion within the long arm of chromosome 5, del(5q), or 5q- occurs in 30% of patients with MDS, 50% of patients with AML arising secondary to MDS or prior chemotherapy, 15% of de novo AMLs, and in only 2% of de novo acute lymphoblastic leukemias (ALLs). The finding of such an abnormality would strongly support a myeloid lineage. Also, recently, the c-Kit protooncogene product may be specific for AML since this expression has not been observed in ALL. Additional cases are needed to support this observation.

ACUTE LYMPHOBLASTIC LEUKEMIA (ALL)

Aplastic/Hypoplastic ALL

Transient pancytopenia and hypoplastic/aplastic bone marrow occurs in a small number of children prior to the onset of ALL. Initially, leukemic blast cells may not be observed. The hypocellular phase is usually followed by apparent bone marrow recovery and later by overt leukemia in weeks or a few months. Contrary to MDS, dysplastic changes are not observed in the hypoplastic state preceding the onset of ALL. Matloub et al. noted that those patients with ALL, after a prolonged period of aplasia, have several common characteristics including female sex; young age; and prevalence of fever, often associated with an infectious disease. Cases have been classified as FAB L1 and are positive for common ALL-associated antigen (CALLA). Cytogenetic studies are too limited to determine whether a pattern exists; however, one child studied in the preleukemic stage revealed numerous chromosomal breaks.

The bone marrow findings preceding ALL have occasionally been interpreted as bone marrow necrosis. Definitive diagnosis is impossible and the marrow should be repeated at a different site or at a later date.

Granular ALL

Granular ALL is a rare morphologic variant of ALL. It is characterized by the presence of more than 5% marrow blasts with at least three clearly defined azurophilic cytoplasmic granules. Both children and adults have the disorder with a low overall incidence (1.8 to 7.6%). The cases are generally associated with a B-cell precursor common phenotype and FAB L2 mor-

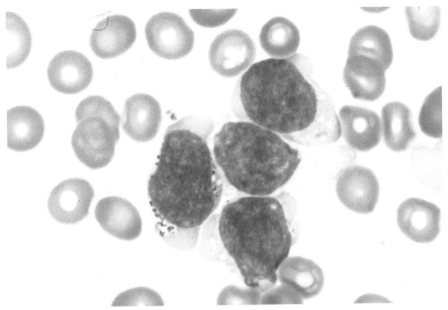

Figure 1.1. Bone marrow showing large type L2 blasts with cytoplasmic granules. This may be confused with acute myeloid leukemia. Granular ALL L2 (×1000). Courtesy of David R. Head.

phology (Fig. 1.1). The granules range from 0.5 to 2 μm in diameter, and occasionally coalesce or aggregate near the Golgi region. They contain small vesicles, electron dense glycogen-like particles, and occasional membranous lamellae and scrolls. The granules resemble immature mast cell-basophil granules, but the relation to mast cells and basophils is unclear at this time. Other cases demonstrate cytoplasmic inclusions ranging from 1.5 to 2.5 μm in diameter that are single membrane bound, and contain slightly electron-dense amorphous material. Some authors have attributed their formation to abnormal mitochondria or fusion of cytoplasmic organelles. Even though granular ALL may represent an entity with poor response to therapy in adults, some authors do not consider the finding of prognostic significance in children. Others, however, have suggested a relationship between granules and worse prognosis. Interestingly, FAB L1 morphology dominated the group, supporting lack of prognostic significance, whereas FAB L2 accounted for most cases with a poorer prognosis. Such a finding suggests that FAB morphology and not the granules dictates prognosis. Since granular lymphoblasts may be confused with myeloblasts, it is most important that we be aware of granular ALL. To make matters more difficult, some of these cases may assume a hand mirror configuration (Fig. 1.2).

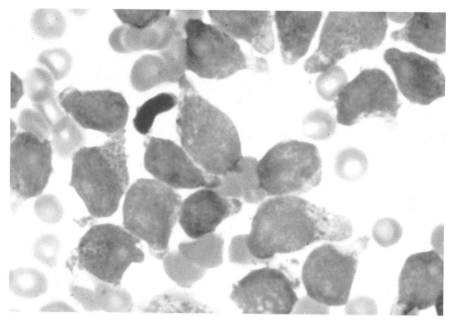

Figure 1.2. Bone marrow showing large type L2 blasts with hand mirror configuration and cytoplasmic granulation. Hand mirror configuration supports lymphoid origin, but may be seen in myeloid leukemias; especially M4 and M5. Granular ALL L2 with hand mirror configuration (×1000). Courtesy of Kathryn Foucar.

ALL—Eosinophilia

Occasionally mild to marked eosinophilia may be observed at diagnosis in ALL. It is important to realize that eosinophilia accompanied by hematological malignancy can be divided into two groups. The myelogenous group includes acute myelomonocytic leukemia with eosinophilia (FAB M4Eo), acute myeloblastic leukemia [FAB M2 t(8;21)] and chronic myelogenous leukemia. In these disorders some of the neoplastic cells appear to differentiate into eosinophils.

To the contrary, in lymphoid malignancies, the transformed tumor cells secrete some eosinophil stimulating cytokines, including interleukin-3, interleukin-5, and granulocyte-macrophage colony-stimulating factor. These cytokines, produced in both FAB L1 and L2 B-lineage ALL, especially with t(5;14)(q31;q32), malignant lymphoma, and adult T-cell lymphoma/leukemia, stimulate the proliferation of normal eosinophilic precursors. Intriguingly, the IgH gene and the interleukin-3 gene are involved in the aforementioned B-lineage ALL translocation. In ALL, the eosinophilia generally resolves with complete remission, but may return with or just prior to relapse (Fig. 1.3).

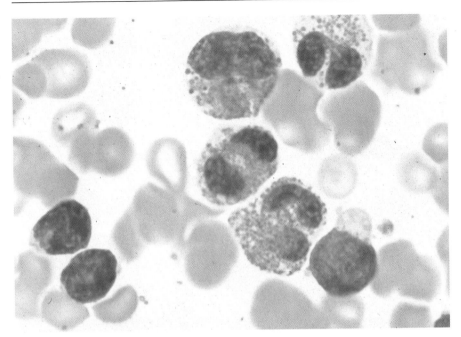

Figure 1.3. Bone marrow demonstrating FAB L1 type lymphoblasts with high nuclear-cytoplasmic ratio. Note presence of large number of eosinophils resulting from cytokines produced by leukemic cells. ALL with eosinophilia (×1000). Courtesy of David R. Head.

In general, when compared to other patients with ALL, those with eosinophilia are old, show greater male predominance, often have evidence of striking organomegaly, and experience an aggressive disease course. The persistent eosinophilia can cause extensive tissue damage, especially involving the heart, lungs, and central nervous system, similar to hypereosinophilic syndrome (HES) and eosinophilic leukemia. All these disorders cause a substantial degree of morbidity and lead to mortality.

Recently, eosinophilia has been associated with cases of T-lymphoblastic lymphoma. These patients were treated and obtained remission, only to relapse later with AML. The karyotypic analysis of the myeloid malignancy revealed a t(8;13)(p11;q11). The authors propose that T-cell lymphoblastic lymphoma with eosinophilia and associated subsequent myeloid malignancy may represent a distinct clinicopathologic entity.

ALL t(4;11)

The t(4;11)(q21;q23) has been associated with marked lineage heterogeneity and with FAB ALL L1, L2 of early B-precursor phenotype, AML FAB M5a, and bilineage-biphenotypic leukemia. Most reported cases have been classified as ALL. The t(4;11) is one of the most common specific chromosomal translocations in ALL, occurring in 2% of childhood and 5% of adult

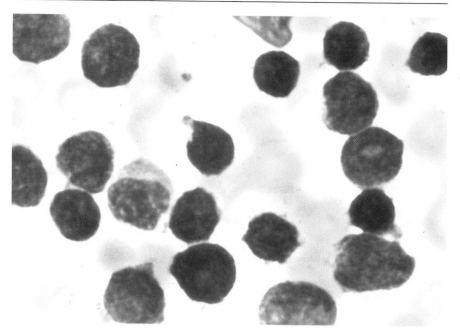

Figure 1.4. Bone marrow showing FAB L1 type blasts from seven month old infant. The cells were CD4, CD19, and TdT positive, but CD10 (CALLA) and HLA-DR negative. ALL with t(4;11) (q21;q23) (×1000). Courtesy of Ralph A. Gruppo.

cases. In childhood ALL, this translocation is associated with the female sex, those less than 1 year old, hepatosplenomegaly, and hyperleukocytosis. There appears to be an age-related difference in treatment outcome. Adults have the worst prognosis, and children 1 to 9 years old appeared to have a better outcome than either infants or adolescents (Fig. 1.4).

Reported cases of AML or a secondary leukemia with t(4;11) have not been well characterized. It is of great interest that virtually all of the reported cases with secondary leukemia had received epipodophyllotoxins or doxorubicin, agents that affect topoisomerase II and are associated with secondary AML characterized by 11q23 abnormalities. For this reason, there has been great interest concerning t(4;11) (q21;q23) because of the demonstration of involvement of the ALL1 (MLL) locus on band 11q23 and of the AF4 locus. A polymerase chain reaction (PCR) has been used on peripheral blood samples to detect the mRNA fusion region for the MLL/AF4 rearrangement, i.e., the molecular equivalent of the t(4;11)(q21;q23) in an early relapsed patient. It was not until 4 weeks later that a blast population with FAB M1 morphology appeared in the bone marrow and the translocation was detected by cytogenetics. Most recently, a monoclonal antibody 7.1, which recognizes the chondroitin sulfate proteoglycan molecule NG2, has been used to screen blast cells from 104 consecutive children initially presenting with ALL. Interestingly, it was found that the blast cell surface expression of NG2 is useful for identifying patients with ALL having t(4;11) or t(11;19).

ALL—Hand Mirror Variant (HMV)

Hand mirror cells (HMC) were first described in 1931 by Lewis in rat lymphocytes. Shortly thereafter, Rich et al. noted HMC in human tissue cultures of normal lymph nodes, infectious mononucleosis, chronic lymphocytic leukemia, and ALL. The HMC were discovered to not only be motile, but also had immunological significance. The uropod (handle) was found to be a specialized area for probing, attaching, endocytosing, and killing.

The first clinical association of HMC to human hematopoietic malignancies was noted by Norberg et al. who observed amoeboid movement configuration (AMC) in cells of patients with acute myelogenous leukemia, lymphosarcoma, and multiple myeloma. Sjögren et al. suggested that finding large numbers of AMC in the bone marrow of children with acute lymphoblastic and myeloblastic leukemia may be indicative of an improved prognosis. Shortly after this report, the term "hand mirror cell" was introduced to replace AMC and was accepted in the medical literature. Additional survival studies performed on children with ALL-HMV revealed variable results. Unfortunately, these cases were not investigated by current technology, which would have allowed more detailed immunophenotypic analysis of the HMC.

Liso et al. and Mazur et al. described a subset of adult ALL-HMV that was similar to the first reported case. This subset revealed female predominance, null phenotype, acid phosphatase and terminal deoxynucleotidyl transferase positivity, indolent course, and poor response to therapy. No sex-age-FAB classification studies were performed on this group to determine ultimate prognosis. Regrettably, none of these cases were studied by means of modern flow cytometric analysis.

Since immune complexes can cause normal lymphocytes to form uropods in vitro, ALL-HMVs were investigated in regard to possible viral stimulation. Although cross reactive immunoglobulins against core proteins of the baboon endogenous and simian sarcoma viruses were detected in bone marrow plasma of ALL-HMV patients, the significance of these findings remains unclear.

Most cases of HMV were initially ALLs with FAB L1, L2, and even L3 classification (Fig. 1.5). Occasionally, AMLs, frequently monocytic, have been reported with HMCs. Most recently, it has been noted that many ALL-HMVs are of mixed lineage and express adhesion molecules (CD2, CD56). These have a propensity for developing extramedullary leukemia, and central nervous system involvement. Therefore, the finding of significant (>30% HMC of the malignant population in the bone marrow) should alert the hematologist/hematopathologist to investigate such cases carefully

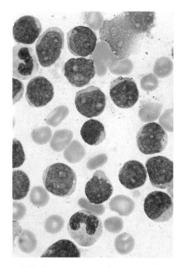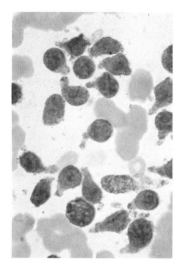

Figure 1.5. Bone marrow from a patient with ALL hand mirror variant. Left panel shows bone marrow directly smeared on slide. Right panel demonstrates marrow collected in EDTA before smearing. Lack of hand mirror configuration in right panel due to chelating effect on cytoskeleton, ALL-hand mirror variant (×400).

to accurately determine pathogenesis, prognosis, and correct therapeutic intervention.

AGGRESSIVE NK CELL LEUKEMIA (ANKCL)

ANKCL is not to be confused with large granular lymphocyte (LGL) leukemia, alias Tγ- lymphoproliferative disease, lymphoproliferative disease of granular lymphocytes, and T-chronic lymphocytic leukemia. LGL leukemia is associated with the clinical syndrome of chronic neutropenia with increased numbers of LGLs in the peripheral blood. It has been recommended that LGL-leukemia be classified into T-LGL leukemia (CD3+), and natural killer-LGL (NK-LGL) leukemia (CD3−). NK-LGL leukemias are clonal, as demonstrated by cytogenetics, but lack convenient clonal markers such as receptor gene rearrangements. These patients are younger than T-LGL leukemic patients; more often have systemic B symptoms; and typically have more massive hepatosplenomegaly, lymphadenopathy, and gastrointestinal tract involvement. Some of these individuals probably overlap with ANKCL cases, and will be more clearly defined as additional information and application of new technology become available.

ANKCL is a clinically aggressive disorder with fever, hepatosplenomegaly, pancytopenia, and abnormal immature lymphoid cells in the peripheral blood and/or bone marrow. The abnormal immature lymphoid cells have a blastic appearance or resemble atypical lymphocytes. Some cases contain abnormal cells that demonstrate clumped nuclear chromatin and a prominent single nucleolus (Fig. 1.6). The cytoplasm is abundant, basophilic, and contains medium to large granules. Interestingly, some show a chronic course before becoming aggressive, suggesting a relation to NK-LGL cases. However, the majority were extremely aggressive, with death occurring within 4 months.

The clinical presentation of NK leukemia is varied and ranges from a chronic indolent course, usually occurring in older patients and compatible with prolonged survival, through transformation from a chronic to an acute lymphoproliferative disease, to an acute presentation and short remission, usually occurring in the younger patient.

Gardiner et al. reported a case of ANKCL in a 5-year-old male child who was initially diagnosed with neuroblastoma. The bone marrow aspirate showed clumps of undifferentiated cells with the following phenotype: CD56 strong+, CD33 weak+, CD45−, CD2−, CD19−, CD16−, and CD57−. Cytochemistry was noncontributory. The patient responded to ALL chemotherapy, but relapsed 4 weeks into treatment and eventually died 25 weeks after initial presentation. The NK cells produced a number of cytokines. Tissue necrosis factor α (TNF-α), interleukin 6 (IL6), IL1Ra, and transforming growth factor-β (TGF-β) were found to be concentrated in the bone marrow in this patient, but not the plasma. TNF-α was present at

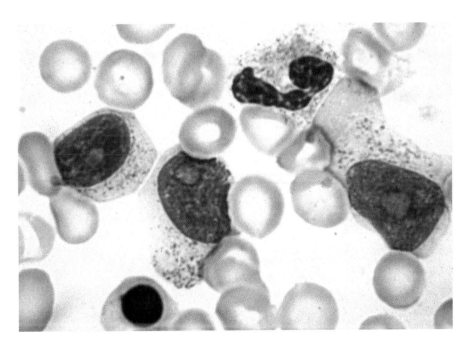

Figure 1.6. Bone marrow from a patient with ANKCL showing large blastic NK cells with prominent nucleoli, clumped nuclear chromatin, and moderate amounts of basophilic cytoplasm containing granules ANKCL ($\times$1000). Courtesy of Nobutaka Imamura.

a high concentration in bone marrow, probably a reflection of the associated disease pathology of severe bone pain and pyrexia. Karyotype of the initial bone marrow aspirate revealed a 46XY t(1;22)(q42;q13) on 12 metaphases, while one metaphase had 47, XY, + iso (9q).

Additional well-documented cases of this disorder need to be reported to increase our understanding of this disease.

ACUTE MYELOID LEUKEMIA (AML)

AML M0

In 1991, the FAB group added an additional FAB subtype that could not be diagnosed by morphology or cytochemical light microscopy criteria alone. This subtype was designated minimally differentiated AML FAB AML M0 (Figs. 1.7 and 1.8). The diagnostic criteria are summarized in Table 1.1. Saito et al. have examined MPEX with antiMPEX monoclonal antibody in four patients by immunohistochemistry and were able to detect 3% or more MPEX positive cells in all cases. They suggested that immunological studies for MPEX by immunohistochemistry may be inexpensive and useful for establishing a diagnosis of FAB M0.

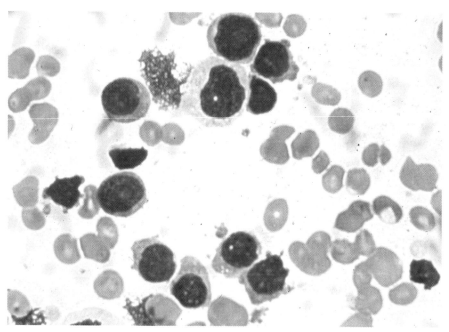

Figure 1.7. Bone marrow demonstrating blasts with oval nuclei, variably prominent nucleoli, moderate basophilic cytoplasm with some cells showing blebbing. FAB AML M0 (×400). Courtesy of Roberto Stasi.

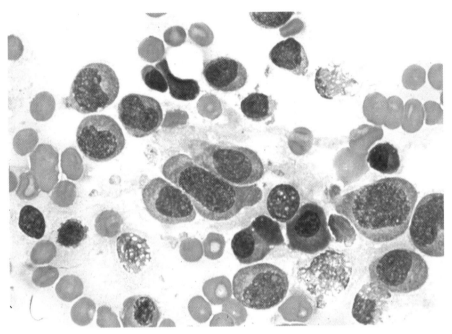

Figure 1.8. Bone marrow from another patient revealing monocytoid features, i.e., indented nuclei, abundant cytoplasm, and prominent Golgi zones. FAB AML M0 with monocytoid features (×400). Courtesy of Roberto Stasi.

FAB M0 occurs in about 5 to 10% of AML cases. FAB M0 is usually associated with those with a higher incidence of prior hematologic disease, low white blood count, few peripheral blood blasts, lower marrow cellularity, and a tendency towards older age. The blast cells usually comprise more than 90% of the bone marrow cells, have fine to slight coarse nuclear chromatin, and contain two to four variably prominent nucleoli. The cytoplasm is pale to slightly basophilic and lacks Auer rods. Rare maturing granulocytes may demonstrate dysplastic features. Virtually all the blast cells are type I. Complex karyotypes have been reported in a large number of cases, but no single chomosomal abnormality has been observed. Nevertheless, t(9;11)(p21;q23) reported in de novo FAB M5 has been observed in FAB M0 and FAB M4 subtypes. Molecular analysis has detected frequent T-cell receptor (TCR) and immunoglobulin gene rearrangements. The above data suggests M0 cells originate from an early hematopoietic precursor that is manifested by a very poor prognosis. Treatment failure is usually due to resistant disease; however, regimens containing vincristine and prednisone showed an advantage. Intriguingly, those AML M0 cases that relapse demonstrate monoblastic or megakaryoblastic lineage. Such a finding suggests that FAB M0 may need to be reclassified as our biotechnology becomes more sophisticated.

Table 1.1
Summary of Diagnostic Features in FAB AML M0[a]

FAB type	Bone marrow	Immunophenotype
AML-M0	≥ 30% blasts	≥20% blasts
	Negative or <3% blasts reactive with MPEX, SBB, or NSE	express one or more myeloid antigens: CD13, CD14, CD33, MPEX
	Electron microscopy (EM) may be positive for MPEX in granules, nuclear envelope, and/or endoplasmic reticulum	Lymphoid antigen blasts (−), but Tdt and CD7 may be (+).

[a]see page 17 for other FAB AMLs.

AML M6-Erythroleukemia

Erythroleukemia constitutes approximately 3% of all cases of acute leukemia and is very rare in children. It represents a heterogeneous group of disorders encompassing chronic erythroleukemia (myelodysplastic disorders), acute leukemias with myeloblastic, proerythroblastic, and mixed leukemic cellular components. The diagnosis of this leukemia, perhaps more than all the others, needs evaluation of many additional cases by modern technology.

The FAB criteria for M6 require that at least 50% of the bone marrow nucleated cells are of erythroid origin and that at least 30% of the nonerythroid cells (NEC) are myeloblasts. If the blast cells are less than 30% of the NEC, a diagnosis of some form of a MDS is considered. This type of leukemia with associated myeloblasts was first described by Di Guglielmo in 1917 and has been referred to as Di Guglielmo's syndrome (M6A) (Fig. 1.9). To further complicate matters, another form of erythroleukemia exists that was described by Di Guglielmo in 1926 that can not be diagnosed by the above FAB criteria. This has been variously referred to as Di Guglielmo's disease, pure erythroleukemia, erythremic myelosis or M6B (Fig. 1.10). Even though the myeloblasts are usually less than 30% of the NEC in pure erythroleukemia (M6B), many hematologists/hematopathologists consider this an acute leukemia by morphology and clinical course. Kowal-Vern et al. believe cases with a preponderance of proerythroblasts should be incorporated into the FAB classification and designated M6B. They suggest the diagnosis of M6B should be established by the finding of >30% proerythroblasts in the BM (determined by dividing the number of proerythroblasts by the total erythroid population). In addition, these authors suggest that mixed erythroleukemias may also exist. The classification of M6A and M6B has recently been accepted by the American Society of Hematopathology and the World Health Organization.

Both of these acute erythroleukemias (M6A, M6B) can be defined on the basis of qualitative and quantitative morphologic findings. They present

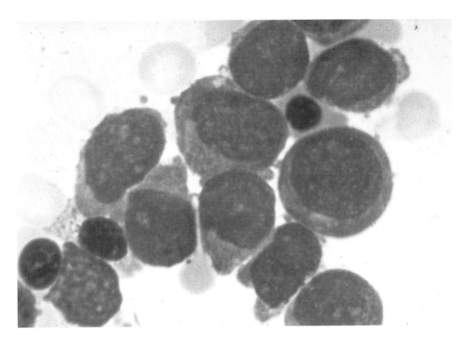

Figure 1.9. Bone marrow from a patient with erythroleukemia. Note prominence of myeloblasts in this particular area of the slide. This meets FAB criteria for M6 and represents Di Guglielmo's syndrome M6A (×1000).

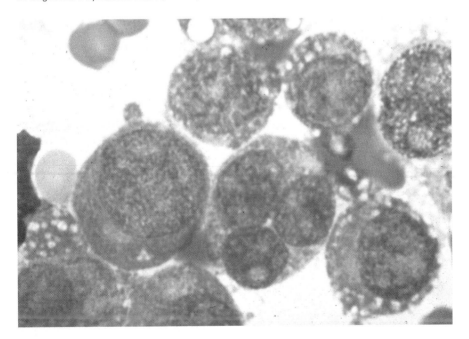

Figure 1.10. Bone marrow showing blasts with large round nuclei, with occasional prominent nucleoli and frequently vacuolated basophilic cytoplasm. Note trinucleated blast. Multinucleated erythroid elements and other myelodysplastic features may be seen in erythroleukemia. Di Guglielmo's disease M6B (×1000).

with leukemic dyserythropoiesis (megaloblastic features, multinucleation, nuclear fragmentation, vacuolated proerythroblasts) and dysmyelopoiesis (abnormal myeloblasts, nuclear/cytoplasmic asynchrony, and Auer rods); however, in pure erythroleukemia (M6B) few to no myeloblasts, no Auer rods, and negative MPEX staining are observed. Strikingly, the malignant proerythroblasts demonstrate coarse (block) PAS positivity, whereas, the more mature precursors usually show diffuse (blush) positivity. Nonspecific esterases may be strongly positive and iron stains frequently reveal ringed sideroblasts. Flow cytometric analysis for glycophorin A, and transmission electron microscopy to demonstrate ferritin rhopheocytosis have been used in some cases to establish lineage and diagnosis.

Cytogenetic analysis has been used to classify subsets of erythroleukemia. Cuneo et al. found that patients with a higher percentage of proerythroblasts/basophilic erythroblasts had a higher incidence of more than two karyotypic abnormalities and a shorter survival. Furthermore, Bernheim et al. observed that increased karyotypic abnormalities correlated with excess of proerythroblasts in their studies. Contrariwise, Olopade et al. found no correlation between morphological features and either cytogenetic abnormalities or clinical outcome. They observed that acute erythroleukemia when defined by FAB morphologic criteria consists of two distinct groups: one group tends to be older with complex cytogenetic abnormalities, especially of chromosomes 5 and/or 7, and shares biologic and clinical features with treated AML; the other group, with simple or no detectable cytogenetic abnormalities, has a more favorable prognosis when treated with intensive chemotherapy. Finally, Davey et al. in an analysis of 52 patients with erythroleukemia divided them into two groups on the basis of the percentage of proerythroblasts and basophilic erythroblasts, concluded that the morphology of erythroblasts in patients with AML M6 may correlate with cytogenetic abnormalities and rate of complete remission. Additional confusion has been created by cases of AML in which the leukemic cells appear to be undifferentiated blasts by light microscopy; however, further analysis by immunologic markers or ultrastructural studies reveal these cells to be very primitive erythroid cells. Some investigators believe these cases should be classified as M6.

Acute Basophilic Leukemia (ABL)

Basophilic leukemia (BL) is a rare heterogeneous disorder that may occur in the chronic phase of chronic myelogenous leukemia (CML) or as a manifestation of the accelerated phase of CML. In addition, it may present as a Ph^1—negative, leukocyte alkaline phosphatase (LAP) positive de novo chronic leukemia. Basophilia has been associated with AMLs with t(6;9), t(3;6) and inv(16) chromosomal abnormalities. The AML M2 baso variant associated with t(6;9)(p23;q34), has been characterized by granulocytic maturation and a variable infiltrate of blast cells with basophilic granules. The involved genes have been cloned and named *DEK* (on chromosome 6) and *CAN* (on chromosome 9). The product derived from the fusion gene p165$^{DEK-CAN}$ protein is involved in the control of DNA transcription. Of interest is the finding that the translocation may be present in AML M1, M4, MDSs and acute myelofibrosis and not always linked with basophil precursors. Such findings have suggested that AMLs with t(6;9) display multilineage myelodysplasia resulting in neoplasias evolving from the myeloid stem cell.

De novo acute basophilic leukemia is an uncommon variant of acute non-lymphocytic leukemia. It is usually characterized by a very rapid clinical course with symptoms of hyperhistaminemia, peptic ulceration, gastrointestinal and cerebrovascular bleeding, and resistance to therapy. Leukocyte counts vary, and most patients have anemia and thrombocytopenia. Some patients have developed anaphylactoid reactions and disseminated intravascular coagulation (DIC) with massive hemorrhage following treatment. Such life threatening events have been shown to be secondary to tumor lysis (basophilic degranulation) rather than to mast cell mediated anaphylactic reaction to drug therapy. This interpretation was supported in some cases by demonstration of heparin release from the basophilic blast granules.

Blood and bone marrow contain agranular blasts that may resemble myeloblasts or lymphoblasts. The nuclei may be lobulated or indented with prominent nucleoli. The cytoplasm may be intensely basophilic and may either lack or show basophilic granules (Fig. 1.11). The marrow is generally hypercellular with a moderate increase in reticulum fibers.

Basophilic leukemic cells are MPEX negative, but toluidine blue or Astra blue positive. Rarely, TdT positive blasts have been reported. Cytogenetic findings have revealed a heterogeneous karyotype analysis. Ultrastructural studies demonstrated blasts with considerable nuclear/cytoplasmic variability. The basophilic granules also varied markedly from case to case. Some, but not all cases demonstrate the theta granule.

AML M1, M0, AUL, and ALL must be distinguished from ABL; however, this is not always possible by routine cytochemical stains and immunologic markers. Indeed, ultrastructural analysis may be the court of final appeal in establishing the diagnosis. Cases of so called basophilic leukemia with t(9;22) represent an accelerated phase or blast crisis of CML which may be the initial event of this disorder. Since CML represents a pluripotent stem cell disorder and ABL exemplifies a predominant disorder of basophilic lineage, one must question the veracity of classifying blast crisis in the former as an acute basophilic leukemia without emphasizing the origin (Fig. 1.12).

Eosinophilic Leukemia (EL)/Hypereosinophilic Syndrome (HES)

Eosinophilic leukemia is a rare, poorly defined disorder that may present with a marked proliferation of mature eosinophils and a small increase of blasts that make it difficult to distinguish from other conditions, especially

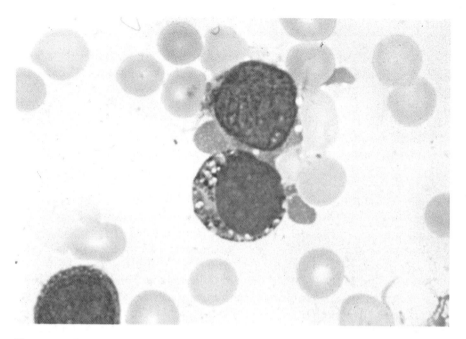

Figure 1.11. Bone marrow showing basophilic blasts. Note one is granular and vacuolated. The other does not reveal prominent granulation. Acute basophilic leukemia (×1000). Courtesy of Robert McKenna.

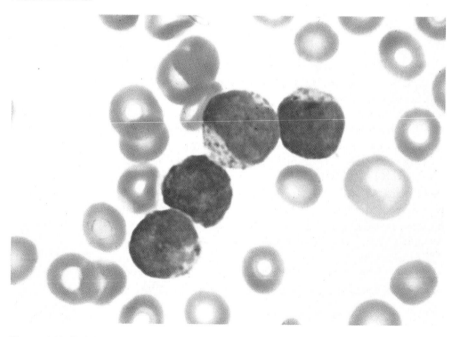

Figure 1.12. Peripheral blood from patient with a basophilic blast crisis of CML. Note numerous blast cells showing basophilic granules. Basophilic blast crisis of CML (×1000). Courtesy of Dan Pankowsky.

the HES. HES is defined as a persistent unexplained eosinophilia of $1.5 \times 10^9/L$ or greater for 6 months or longer or death before 6 months associated with signs and symptoms of this disorder. This conundrum exists because morphological findings and clinical manifestations can be very similar. The damage of organs (i.e., heart, central nervous system, lungs, and skin) results from the proteins produced by the eosinophilic granules; whether benign or neoplastic. Patients demonstrate evidence of congestive heart failure, new heart murmurs, and/or conduction defects and arrhythmias. Interstitial pulmonary infiltrates and pleural effusion may occur. Nervous system dysfunction may be profound. Others have reported cytogenetic abnormalities in HES; however, Fauci et al. proposed empirical criteria for diagnosing HES and identified three groups of patients with different clinical courses. The initial group was asymptomatic with a favorable course; the second group was symptomatic with some organ involvement and a more serious prognosis. Finally, the third group manifested hepatosplenomegaly with early treatment-induced anemia and thrombocytopenia. This latter group demonstrated cytogenetic alterations and blastic crisis evolution consistent with an aggressive form of leukemia. Even though blast transformation is the cornerstone for evidence of leukemia, the presence of immature cells of the granulocytic series in the blood is not, in itself, sufficient for a diagnosis of leukemia. Therefore, in the absence of a clonal chromosome abnormality such cases should be relegated to the HES, unless the marrow and other organs are infiltrated with eosinophilic blast cells.

Both EL and HES may reveal leukocyte counts well over $20 \times 10^9/L$ and absolute eosinophil counts greater than $1.5 \times 10^9/L$ sustained for 6 months. The eosinophils manifest a wide spectrum of morphologic changes including nuclear hypo/hypersegmentation, hypogranulation, and cytoplasmic vacuolization (Fig. 1.13). Myeloblasts may occasionally be present in the peripheral blood in HES. Bone marrow of EL and HES show hypercellularity, marked increase in eosinophils in all stages of development, increased myeloblasts, promyelocytes, and dysgranulopoiesis (Fig. 1.14). Progression leads to increased numbers of blasts and immature granulocytic precursors; more myelodysplasia and fibrosis. Other laboratory findings, usually associated with CML, such as hyperuricemia, elevated B12 levels, and occasionally decreased leukocyte alkaline phosphatase determination may be observed. Cases with eosinophilia that are $Ph^1 +$ should be classified as a variant of CML. Also, a chronic eosinophilic leukemia exists that is associated with more maturing eosinophilic forms and a longer clinical course (Fig. 1.15).

Transmission electron microscopy of both EL and HES reveals homogeneous granules within the eosinophils in contrast to the normal crystalline structure.

Cytogenetic abnormalities support a diagnosis of EL rather than HES. Trisomy 7, 8, 17+, 12p13, 5q31, t(2;5)(p23;q35) and chromosomal aneu-

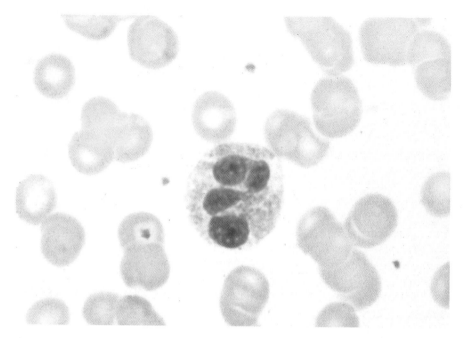

Figure 1.13. Peripheral blood from a patient with acute eosinophilic leukemia. Hypersegmented eosinophil with maldistribution of granules. Acute eosinophilic leukemia (×1000).

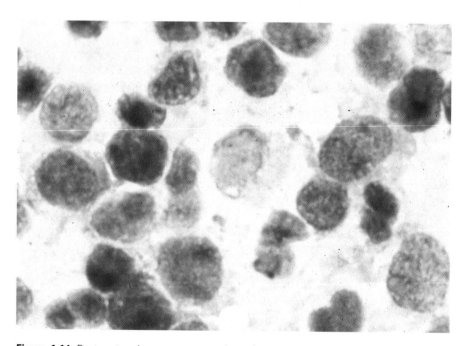

Figure 1.14. Postmortem bone marrow specimen from same patient in Figure 1.13. Unfortunately an antemortem marrow was not performed; however, large mononuclear cells that appeared to be blasts were noted. Tissues throughout body were heavily infiltrated with eosinophils, eosinophilic precursors, and blasts. Acute eosinophilic leukemia (×400).

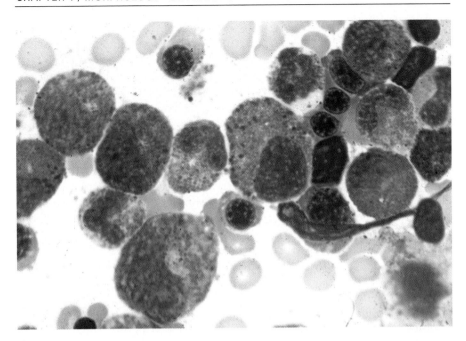

Figure 1.15. Bone marrow from a patient with chronic eosinophilic leukemia. Eosinophils in various stages of development. Some show basophilic granules. Chronic eosinophilic leukemia (× 1000). Courtesy of Brian Kueck.

ploidy have been reported in some cases of EL. The demonstration of a clonal cytogenetic abnormality is now considered confirmatory of leukemia. In support of this concept, cases of HES without karyotypic abnormalities developed a malignant clone 46, XY, t(5;11)(p15;q13) and underwent malignant transformation to an acute EL.

Treatment should be directed at reducing the eosinophil count in order to obviate the toxic effects of the products of the eosinophilic granules. Steroids, hydroxyurea, and vincristine have been used in HES with multiagent drugs utilized in more aggressive cases. Prognosis is very poor in acute EL.

Hypocellular AML

Hypocellular AML (HAML) and MDS are conditions in which the bone marrow cellularity is less than 30%. In calculating the percentage of bone marrow cellularity, hematopoietic cell volume should be compared with total bone marrow space, with the fibrotic area being excluded from this calculation. The blast percentage in the bone marrow and/or blood is 30% or more in HAML and less than 30% in MDS. Approximately 5% of adult patients presenting with AML have hypocellular bone marrow biopsies. This finding is more common in older adults, probably due to fact that some of these start as hypocellular MDS. The majority of these patients are pancytopenic and occasional blasts may be found in the peripheral blood. The FAB classification is usually AML M0, M1, or M2.

Hypocellular AML needs to be distinguished from hypocellular MDS and aplastic anemia. Hypocellular MDS usually presents with increased reticulin and foci of blasts (less than 30%). Nests of nonparatrabecular myeloblasts termed abnormal localization of immature precursors (ALIPs) may be observed. In aplastic anemia, however, the normal hematopoietic marrow is replaced by fat spaces; reticulin is not increased; and nonhematopoietic cells, lymphocytes, plasma cells, and macrophages remain in normal distribution.

At times, however, separating hypocellular MDS from aplastic anemia may be extremely perplexing. Appelbaum et al. suggested that a clonal cytogenetic abnormality in aplastic anemia is an indication of an MDS. They studied 183 patients with aplastic anemia and noted that only 7 (4%) showed clonal chromosomal abnormalities (5q-, monosomy 7, trisomy 8) frequently seen in MDS or AML. Although five patients (3%) had no cytogenetic abnormalities and subsequently developed either MDS or leukemia, they concluded that all patients with aplastic anemia may have some risk of developing leukemia. Nevertheless, they added that those with cytogenetic abnormalities are at an especially high risk. In contrast, Moormeir et al. noted three patients with hypocellular marrow, mild dysplasia, and trisomy 6 who did not have the clinical characteristics of MDS. Furthermore, two of the three patients responded to treatment directed at autoimmune-mediated aplastic anemia; however, some MDS patients have responded to antithymocyte globulin (ATG). Such findings suggest that all clonal cytogenetic abnormalities may not be a specific indicator of MDS or AML and that response to ATG does not clearly establish the diagnosis; however, the finding of an abnormality common to MDS or AML such as -5, del(5q), 7, del(7q) and trisomy 8 would support a premalignant myeloid proliferation. Recently, some HAML patients have achieved complete hematological reconstitution following granulocyte-stimulating factor therapy.

CD7 Positive AML

Conflicting results exist regarding the prognostic importance of CD7 expression in AML. Differences in the method of determining CD7 positivity, the antibody used, the therapy administered, and the CD7 level used as a cut-off point to reduce it to a binary variable have all been postulated to account for the discordant findings. CD7 is expressed in approximately 10 to 30% of AML patients with FAB M0, M1, and M5a predominately. Such cases are associated with immature markers such as HLA-DR, CD34, and TdT. Some investigators attribute adverse prognostic significance to CD7+AML, others found no difference in outcome between CD7+AML and CD7-AML. Also, some investigators found differences in age and sex; whereas others found no differences.

AML 3(q21;q26)

AMLs or MDSs presenting with the chromosome abnormality 3(q21;q26) have been associated with normal platelet counts or thrombocytosis, increased megakaryocytes, micromegakaryocytes, and unfavorable prognosis. The platelet counts can exceed 1000×10^9/L.

The classification of these AMLs have been difficult and FAB M1, FAB M6 and FAB M4 have been reported. Grigg et al. evaluated 1200 cases with clonal cytogenetic abnormalities and found 24 patients with a 3q rearrangement at q21 and q25-26. Thirteen patients presented with de novo AML, 10 with myelodysplasia, and 1 in blast crisis of CML. Twenty patients (83%) had megakaryocytic dysplasia and 14 (58%) had normal or increased numbers of megakaryocytes, but only four patients (16%) had absolute thrombocytosis $>500 \times 10^9$/L. Further review by this group of AML cases revealed that a platelet count $>500 \times 10^9$/L at presentation was highly suggestive of an underlying 3q abnormality. Also, 15 to 20% of patients with a 3q abnormality will have thrombocytosis.

Additional cases involving 3q25 have been described. Two cases were FAB M2 and one a CML in blast crisis. All three cases demonstrated identical t(2;3)(p13;q26) abnormalities. Interestingly, they showed no decrease of blood thrombocytes, dysplastic megakaryocytes, short remission, and unfavorable course of disease. Therefore, the clinical and morphological findings in patients with the t(2;3)(p13;q26) resembled the above cases with 3q21q26 syndromes or with other chromosome rearrangements involving 3q21 or 3q26. In general, the response of these patients to conventional antileukemia therapy is uniformly poor, despite hematological and clinical differences between the subtypes of 3q rearrangements.

Other translocations, t(3;5)(q25.1;q34), have been associated with AML with involvement of granulocytes, megakaryocytes, and erythroid precursors. Such a translocation has been associated with both MDS and AML.

Myeloid/NK-Leukemia

This unique subset of acute leukemia has recently been described and has diagnostic importance in regard to correct therapy. The malignant cells in the majority of cases revealed deeply invaginated nuclear membranes, scant cytoplasm with fine azurophilic granularity, and finely granular Sudan black B and MPEX cytochemical reactivity. These findings were remarkably similar to acute promyelocytic leukemia (FAB AML M3); particularly the microgranular variant (FAB AML M3v) (Figs. 1.16 and 1.17). Scott et al. evaluated 350 consecutive cases of de novo AML and identified 20 cases (6%) that belonged to this unique subtype. Interestingly, such cases share features of both myeloid and NK cells. Despite the striking resemblance to acute promyelocytic leukemia, all 20 cases lacked the t(15;17) and 17 cases tested lacked the promyelocytic/retinoic acid receptor alpha (RAR alpha) fusion transcript in RT-PCR assays. None of the leukemic cells of these cases was able to differentiate in vitro in response to all-transretinoic acid (ATRA), suggesting that these cases may account for some mistakenly diagnosed acute promyelocytic leukemias that have not shown a clinical response to

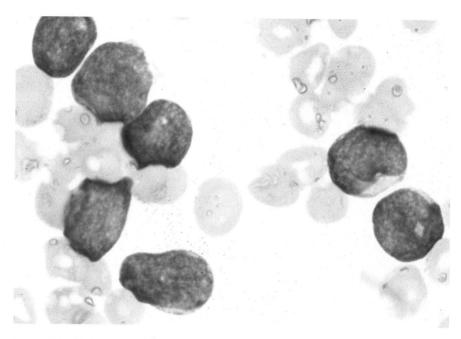

Figure 1.16. Peripheral blood from a patient with myeloid/NK acute leukemia. Note blast cells with scanty cytoplasm. Granules are difficult to discern similar to FAB AML M3v. Note notched nucleus in one of the blasts. Myeloid/NK acute leukemia (× 1000). Courtesy of David R. Head.

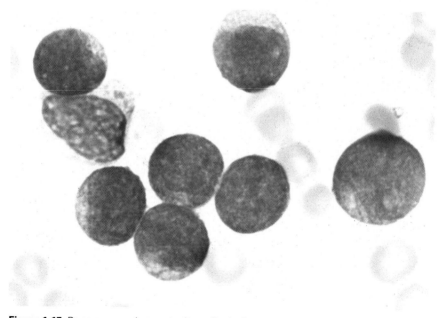

Figure 1.17. Bone marrow demonstrating cells similar to those in peripheral blood. Some of the cells show notched nuclei and granules in the cytoplasm. Myeloid/NK acute leukemia (× 1000). Courtesy of David R. Head.

ATRA. Therefore, recognition of this entity will be important in distinguishing these ATRA-nonresponsive cases from ATRA-responsive true acute promyelocytic leukemia. Recently, Kaya et al. described a patient with myeloma treated with combination chemotherapy who, 3 years later, developed a myeloid/NK acute leukemia. The patient was treated with low-dose etoposide and obtained a complete remission; however, the myeloma recurred and responded to dexamethasone and low dose etoposide. Unfortunately, the leukemia recurred, etoposide produced a severe myelosuppression and the patient died of sepsis.

BILINEAGE/BIPHENOTYPIC ACUTE LEUKEMIA

There is considerable confusion over terminology involving acute leukemias with blast cells that express characteristics of more than one hematopoietic lineage. This confusion is compounded by disagreement on the constitution of adequate evidence for lineage commitment. Furthermore, information is limited as to the sequence or concentration of surface antigens on normal hematopoietic precursor cells and on leukemic blasts. Acute leukemias with blast cells that express characteristics of more than one hematopoietic lineage have been assigned numerous names. These designations include biphenotypic, bilineal, hybrid, biclonal, chimeric, mixed, simultaneous, synchronous, metachronous, and lineage switch. In addition to the confusion in terminology, there is lack of agreement on the criteria to be adapted for adequate identification and classification. Accepted criteria for diagnosis and a standard terminology are definitely needed. Interestingly, HMCs and adhesive molecules have been associated with biphenotypic leukemia (Fig. 1.18).

The most important and useful discrimination that has to be made is between biphenotypic and bilineal acute leukemia. Biphenotypic or acute mixed lineage leukemia should be confined to cases where coexpression of lymphoid and myeloid markers occur on the same cells. Bilineal leukemia represents those cases in which two separate blast populations exist; one showing myeloid features, and the other displaying lymphoid characteristics. Bilineal leukemias can be synchronous (leukemias in which there are simultaneous, distinct populations of leukemic cells of more than one lineage) or metachronous (in which one lineage is expressed following the other). Metachronous leukemia is a recurrence of the original leukemic clone with changes in the cellular expression to include new antigens or gene rearrangements associated with another lineage. In order to separate these cases from therapy-induced, second malignancies, the reappearance of the original clone must be demonstrated by the presence of common cytogenetic abnormalities or identical gene rearrangements.

Antigenic asynchrony is described as a situation in which the leukemic cell coexpresses early and late differentiation antigens in combinations not found on normal differentiating cells. Such expression has been found in T-lineage lymphoblastic leukemia and some cases of acute myeloblastic leukemia.

The frequency of ectopic antigen expression in acute leukemia is ex-

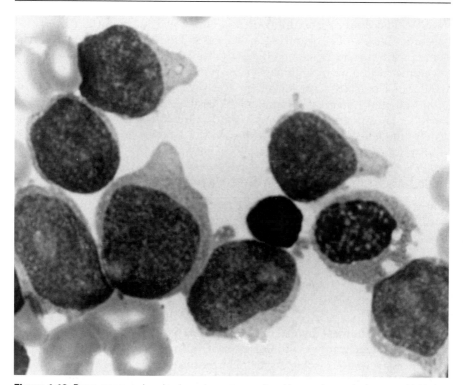

Figure 1.18. Bone marrow showing large immature cells with prominent single- to multiple- nucleoli and moderately abundant basophilic cytoplasm with occasional budding and hand mirror configuration. Immunophenotypic analysis revealed the cells marked as myeloid (CD13, CD33) and T-cells (CD2, CD5, CD7). They were also CD34 and TdT positive. They fulfilled the Catovsky criteria for biphenotypic acute leukemia (×1000).

tremely variable due to the panel of antibodies measured, interpretation, and technology. Reports in the literature for the presence of lymphoid-associated antigens in AML ranged from 2 to 60% of cases, whereas, myeloid antigen expression in ALL appears to vary with age, approaching 35% in adults and ranging from 3.5 to 20% in childhood. Del Vecchio et al. observed that 92% of acute leukemias expressed single-lineage features or only one ectopic marker on their blasts. Biphenotypic leukemias accounted for 5% of the entire series.

Cytogenetic studies have identified karyotypes that are more frequently associated with biphenotypic leukemias. They include t(9;22) aberrations of chromosome 11 at band 23, chromosome 14 at band q32, and trisomy 13. Such abnormalities support the concept that biphenotypic and bilineal acute leukemias arise from a multipotent stem cell with early maturation arrest.

Another phenomenon that requires comment is lineage switch. This involves the expression of markers of one lineage at diagnosis with a "switch" to a different phenotype or lineage at the time of relapse. This has been reported in children with leukemia of the T-cell subtype in which relapse occurred as AML or myelomonocytic leukemia. Interestingly, karyotypic analysis in such cases has revealed that chromosome 11, region 11q23 is most commonly involved.

As increasing numbers of bilineal/biphenotypic acute leukemias are studied, we should gain greater insight into designing specific therapeutic regimens. It is already known that some of these hybrid patterns have distinct clinical features at the time of presentation and poor response to treatment. More information is needed at this juncture to enable us to deal with these leukemias more effectively.

The morphological findings, comments, and references for each of the above leukemias are summarized in Table 1.2.

Table 1.2
Summary of Morphology

Diagnosis FAB Subtype	Morphology	Comment	References
AUL	Agranular type 1 blasts Nuclear chromatin fine Two to four variably prominent nuclei Auer rods absent Cytoplasm pale to slightly basophilic	Fewer cases will be reported as more sophisticated biotechnology becomes available	Leukemia 1990;4:620–624
Hypocellular/ aplastic ALL	FAB L1 morphology Bone marrow occasionally necrotic	Dysplastic changes not seen in hypoplastic state before ALL	Cancer 1993;71:264–268
Granular ALL	FAB L1 and L2 morphology seen Granules range from 0.5 to 0.5 to 2 μm in diameter and may resemble mast cell basophil granules	Importance is that these cases should not be confused with AML	Ann Hematol 1993;67:301–303
ALL with eosinophils	Normal eosinophils and eosinophilic precursors	Eosinophilia result of tumor secreted cytokines ALL t(5;14)(q31;q32) associated with eosinophilia	J Clin Oncol 1987;5:382–390
Acute leukemia with t(4;11)	May have L1, L2, or AUL morphology	Associated with marked lineage heterogeneity. L1, L2 early B-precursor, AML M5a, bilineage-biphenotypic leukemia	Blood 1986;67:689–697

(Continued)

Table 1.2   (Continued)

Diagnosis FAB Subtype	Morphology	Comment	References
Acute leukemia hand mirror variant (ALL-HMV)	Hand mirror shaped cells L1, L2, L3, AML 4, 5 morphology	Recent studies indicate many ALL-HMV are mixed lineage leukemias with adhesive molecules	Hematopathol Mol Hematol 1996; 10:85–98
Aggressive natural killer cell leukemia (ANKCL)	Oval nucleus with clumped nuclear chromatin, prominent single nucleolus, abundant basophilic cytoplasm with medium to large granules	Aggressive disorder with fever, hepato-splenomegaly, pancytopenia, and abnormal lymphoid cells in peripheral blood and/or bone marrow	Br J Haematol 1990;75:49–59
AML-M0	Round to oval nucleus sometimes monocytoid Two to four variably prominent nucleoli Moderate to abundant Pale to slightly basophilic cytoplasm	Requires immunological studies and/or EM-MPEX	Blood 1987;70:1400–1406
AML 6A, 6B Erythroleukemia	AML-6A greater than 50% erythroid with myeloblasts AML-6B greater than 50% erythroid with proerythroblasts	Heterogeneous disorder Also, mixed AML M6C exists Prognosis different for three groups	Am J Clin Pathol 1992;98:34–40
Acute basophilic leukemia (ABL)	Blasts may resemble myeloblasts or lymphoblasts Nuclei may be lobulated, indented with prominent nucleoli Cytoplasm may be intensely basophilic with or without basophilic granules	Must be distinguished from AML M0, M1, AUL, and ALL Distinction may not be possible by cytochemistry and immunological markers EM needed as definitive evidence in some cases	Am J Clin Pathol 1991;96:160–170
Eosinophilic leukemia (EL) Hypereosinophilic syndrome (HES)	Eosinophils manifest a wide spectrum of morphologic changes including nuclear hypo-hypersegmentation, hypogranulation and cytoplasmic vacuolization. EM reveals homogeneous and abnormal crystalline structure within the granules	EL and HES may be extremely difficult to separate Cytogenetic abnormalities and demonstration of clonality support EL	Ann Int Med 1982;97:78–92

Table 1.2   (*Continued*)

Diagnosis FAB Subtype	Morphology	Comment	References
Hypocellular AML	FAB M0, M1, M2 morphology	Needs to be distinguished from hypocellular MDS and aplastic anemia Approximately 5% of adults with AML have hypocellular bone marrow biopsies	Hematol Oncol 1986;4:291–305
CD7 positive AML	FAB M0, M1, M5a predominately	Variable outcomes Needs re-evaluation	Hematopathol Mol Hematol 1996;10:1–38
AML 3(q21;q26)	FAB M1, M4, M6 have been reported	Usually associated with abnormalities in megakaryocytopoiesis	Br J Haematol 1993;83:158–165
Myeloid/NK leukemia	FAB M3; especially the microgranular variant FAB M3v	Show features of myeloid and NK cells Confused with M3 and do all respond to all trans retinoic acid (ATRA)	Blood 1994;84:244–255
Biphenotypic bilineage acute leukemia	Biphenotypic-lymphoid/myeloid variability Bilineal—separate lymphoid/ myeloid population Hand mirror configuration	Confused area. Needs scoring system for reliability	Leuk Lymphoma 1994;13(1):11–14

BIBLIOGRAPHY

Articles

Abruzzo LV, Jaffe ES, Cotelingam JD, et al. T-cell lymphoblastic lymphoma with eosinophilia associated with subsequent myeloid malignancy. Am J Surg Pathol 1992;16:236–245.

Appelbaum FR, Barall J, Storb R, et al. Clonal cytogenetic abnormalities in patients with otherwise typical aplastic anemia. Exp Hematol 1987;15:1134–1139.

Behm FG, Smith FO, Raimondi SC, et al. Human homologue of the rat chondroitin sulfate proteoglycan NG2 detected by monoclonal antibody 7.1, identifies childhood acute lymphoblastic leukemias with t(4;11)(q21;q23) or t(11;19)(q23;p13) and MLL gene rearrangements. Blood 1996;87:1134–1139.

Bennett JM, Catovsky D, Daniel MT, et al. A variant form of acute hypergranular promyelocytic leukemia (M3). Br J Haematol 44:169–170, 1980.

Bennett JM, Catovsky D, Daniel MT, et al. The morphological classification of acute lymphoblastic leukemia: concordance among observers and clinical correlations. Br J Haematol 1981;47:553–561.

Bernheim A, Berger R, Daniel MT, et al. Malignant and reactive erythroblasts in erythroleukemia (M6). Cancer Genet Cytogenet 1983;10:1–10.

Blutters-Sawatzaki R, Borkhardt A, Grathwohl J, et al. Secondary acute myeloid leukemia with translocation (4;11) and MLL/AF4 rearrangement in a 15-year-old boy treated for common acute lymphoblastic leukemia 11 years earlier. Ann Hematol 1995;70:31–35.

Buhring HJ, Ullrich A, Schaudt K, et al. The product of the proto-oncogene c-Kit p145/{c-Kit} is a human bone marrow surface antigen of hemopoietic precursor cells which is expressed on a subset of acute nonlymphoblastic leukemic cells. Leukemia 1991;5:854–860.

Cuneo A, VanOrshoven A, Michaux JL, et al. Morphologic, immunologic, and cytogenetic studies in erythroleukemia: evidence for multilineage involvement and identification of two distinct cytogenetic-clinicopathological types. Br J Haematol 1990;75:346–354.

Darbyshire PJ, Lilleyman JS. Granular acute lymphoblastic leukemia of childhood: a morphological phenomenon. J Clin Pathol. 1987;40:251–253.

Davey FR, Abraham N Jr, Brunnetto VL. Morphologic characteristics of erythroleukemia (acute myeloid leukemia; FAB-M6): a CALGB study. Am J Hematol 1995;49:29–38.

DelVecchio L, Schiavone EM, Ferrara F, et al. Immunodiagnosis of acute leukemia displaying ectopic antigens: proposal for a classification of promiscuous phenotypes. Am J Hematol 1989;31:173–180.

Fleischman EW, Volkova MA, Frenkel MA, et al. Translocation (2;3)(p13;q26) in two cases of myeloid malignancies. Acute myeloblastic leukemia (M2) and blastic phase of chronic myeloid leukemia. Cancer Genet Cytogenet 1996;87:182–184.

Fradera J, Velez-Garcia E, White JG. Acute lymphoblastic leukemia with unusual cytoplasmic granulation: a morphologic, cytochemical, and ultrastructural study. Blood 1986;68:406–411.

Gardiner CM, Reen DJ, O'Meara A. Recognition of unusual presentation of natural killer cell leukemia. Am J Hematol 1995;50:133–139.

Gu Y, Nakamura T, Alder H, et al. The t(4;11) chromosome translocation of human acute leukemias fuses ALL-1 gene related to Drosophilias trithorax to the AF-4 gene. Cell 1992;71:701–708.

Huang CS, Gomez GA, Kohno SI, et al. Chromosomes and causation of human cancer and leukemia. XXXIV A case of "hypereosinophilic syndrome" with unusual cytogenetic findings in a chloroma, terminating in blastic transformation and CNS leukemia. Cancer 1979;44(4):1284–1289.

Inhorn KC, Aster JC, Roach SA, et al. A syndrome of lymphoblastic lymphoma, eosinophilia, and myeloid hyperplasia/malignancy associated with t(8;13) (p11;q11): description of a distinctive clinicopathologic entity. Blood 1995;85:1881–1887.

Kaya H, Nakamura S, Yamazaki H, et al. Secondary myeloid/natural killer cell acute leukemia appeared in multiple myeloma treated with melphalan. Jap J Clin Hematol 1995;36:682–686.

Keene P, Mendelow B, Pinto MR, et al. Abnormalities of chromosome 12p31 and malignant proliferation of eosinophils: a random association. Br J Haematol 1987;67:25–31.

Kovarik P, Shrit MA, Yuen B, et al. Hand mirror variant of acute lymphoblastic leukemia. Evidence of a mixed leukemia. Am J Clin Pathol. 1992;98:526–530.

Kueck BD, Smith RE, Parkin J, et al. Eosinophilic leukemia: a myeloproliferative disorder distinct from the hypereosinophilic syndrome. Hematol Pathol. 1991; 5:195–205.

Lawlor E, McCann SR, Willoughby R, et al. Basophilic differentiation in Ph-positive blast cell leukemia (letter). Br J Haematol 1983;54:157–160.

Lewis WH. Locomotion of lymphocytes. Bull Johns Hopkins Hosp 1931;49:29–36.

Matutes E, Catovsky D. The value of scoring systems for the diagnosis of biphenotypic leukemia and mature B-cell disorders. Leuk Lymphoma 1994;13 (1):11–14.

Maubach PA, Bauchinger M, Emmerich B, et al. Trisomy 7 and 8 in Ph-negative chronic eosinophilic leukemia. Cancer Genet Cytogenet 1985;17(2):159–164.

Moormeier JA, Rubin CM, LeBeau M, et al. Trisomy 6: a recurring cytogenetic abnormality associated with marrow hypoplasia. Blood 1991;77:1397–1398.

Morishita K, Parganas E, Williams CL, et al. Activation of EVI 1 gene expression in human acute myelogenous leukemia by translocations spanning 300 to 400 kilobases on chromosome band 3q26. Proc Natl Acad Sci USA 1992;89:3937–3941.

Niebrugge DJ, Benjamin DR. Bone marrow necrosis preceding acute lymphoblastic leukemia in childhood. Cancer 1983;52:2162–2164.

Norberg B, Rydgren L, Stenstam M. Amoeboid movement configuration: a cell configuration observed in tumor cells from three cases of bone marrow neoplasia. Scand J Haematol 1974;13:294–304.

Olopade OI, Thangavelu MT, Larson RA, et al. Clinical, morphologic and cytogenetic characteristics of 26 patients with acute erythroblastic leukemia. Blood 1992;80:2873–2882.

Parreira L, Tavares de Castro J, Hibbin JA, et al. Chromosome and cell culture studies in eosinophilic leukaemia. Br J Haematol 1986;62(4):659–669.

Rich AR, Wintrobe MD, Lewis WH. Differentiation of myeloblasts from lymphoblasts by their manner of locomotion: a motion picture study of cells of normal bone marrow, lymph nodes and of leukemic blood. Bull Johns Hopkins Hosp 1939;65:291–309.

Saito M, Kuriyama K, Nagai K, et al. Immunocytochemistry in the diagnosis of acute myeloid leukemia. Jpn J Clin Hematol 1994;35:1297–1304.

Sandoval C, Head DR, Mirro J Jr, et al. Translocation t(9;11)(p21;q23) in pediatric de novo and secondary acute myeloblastic leukemia. Leukemia 1992;6:513–519.

Sato H, Saito H, Ikebuchi K, et al. Biological characteristics of chronic eosinophilic leukemia cells with a t(1;5)(p23;q35) translocation. Leuk Lymphoma 1995; 19:499–505.

Schumacher HR, Desai SN, McClain KL, et al. Acute lymphoblastic leukemia—hand-mirror-variant. Analysis for endogenous retroviral antibodies in bone marrow plasma. Am J Clin Pathol 1989;91:410–416.

Schumacher HR, Perlin E, Miller WM, et al. Hand mirror cell leukemia. Lancet 1977;1:655–656.

Schumacher HR, Skelly ME. Acute basophilic leukemia (letter). Am J Clin Pathol 1992;97:895–896.

Sjögren U, Norberg B, Rydgren L. Amoeboid movement configuration in tumor cells of bone marrow smears from patients with leukemia. Acta Med Scand 1977;201: 381–386.

Soekerman D, VonLindern M, Daenen S, et al. The translocation t(6;9)(p23;q34) shows consistent rearrangement of two genes and defines a myeloproliferative disorder with specific clinical features. Blood 1992;79:2990–2997.

VonLindern M, Fornerod M, Soekermann N, et al. Translocation t(6;9) in acute non-lymphocytic leukemia results in the formation of DEK-CAN fusion gene. Boillere's Clin Hematol 1992;5:857–879.

Yumura-Yagi K, Hara J, et al. Clinical significance of CD7 positive stem cell leukemia. A distinct subtype of mixed lineage leukemia. Cancer 1991;68:2273–2280.

Yates P, Potter MN. Eosinophilic leukemia with an abnormality of 5q 31, the site of the IL5 gene. Clin Lab Haematol 1991;13:211–215.

Yoneda-Kato N, Look AT, Kirstein MN, et al. The t(3;5)(q25.1;q34) of myelodysplastic syndrome and acute myeloid leukemia produces a novel fusion gene, NPM-MLF1. Oncogene 1996;12:265–275.

Yoo TJ, Orman SV, Patil SR, et al. Evolution to eosinophilic leukemia with a t(5:11) translocation in a patient with idiopathic hypereosinophilic syndrome. Cancer Genet Cytogenet 1984;11(4):389–394.

Zucker ML, Plapp FV, Racchel JM, et al. An adult case of acute biphenotypic leukemia with characteristic mixed morphology. Mo Med 1993;90:601–604.

Review Articles

Behm FJ. Morphologic and cytochemical characteristics of childhood lymphoblastic leukemia. Hematol Onc Clin North Am 1990;4:715–741.

Bennett JM, Catovsky D, Daniel MT, et al. Criteria for the diagnosis of acute leukemia of megakaryocytic lineage (M7). Ann Int Med 1985;103:460–462.

Bennett JM, Catovsky D, Daniel MT, et al. Proposal for the recognition of minimally differentiated acute myeloid leukemia. Br J Haematol 1991;78:325–329.

Bennett JM, Catovsky D, Daniel MT, et al. Proposals for the classification of the acute leukemias (FAB Cooperative Group). Br J Haematol 1976;33:451–458.

Bennett JM, Catovsky D, Daniel MT, et al. Proposals for the classification of the myelodysplastic syndromes. Br J Haematol 1982;51:189–199.

Bennett JM, Catovsky D, Daniel MT, et al. Proposed revised criteria for the classification of acute myeloid leukemia. A report of the French-American-British Cooperative Group. Ann Int Med 1985;103:626–629.

Berdeaux DH, Glasser L, Serokmann R, et al. Hypoplastic acute leukemia: review of 70 cases with multivariate regression analysis. Hematol Oncol 1986;4:291–305.

Bernini JC, Timmons CF, Sandler ES. Acute basophilic leukemia in a child. Anaphylactoid reaction and coagulopathy secondary to vincristine-mediated degranulation. Cancer 1995;75:110–114.

Biondi A, Rambaldi A, Rossi V, et al. Detection of ALL-1/AF4 fusion transcript by reverse transcription-polymerase chain reaction for diagnosis and monitoring of acute leukemias with the t(4;11) translocation. Blood 1993;82:2943–2947.

Bittes MA, Neilly ME, LeBeau MM, et al. Rearrangements of chromosome 3 involving bands 3q21 and 3q26 are associated with normal or elevated platelet counts in acute nonlymphocytic leukemia. Blood 1985;66:1362–1370.

Breatnach F, Chessells JM, Greaves MF. The aplastic presentation of childhood leukaemia: a feature of common ALL. Br J Haematol 1981;49:387–393.

Brunning RD, McKenna RW. Atlas of tumor pathology: tumors of the bone marrow, AFIP Fascicle 9. Washington, DC: AFIP, 1994:19–142.

Bruno A, Del Poeta G, Venditti A, et al. Diagnosis of acute myeloid leukemia and system Coulter VCS. Haematologica 1994;79:420–428.

Cadwell FJ, Burns CP, Dick FR, et al. Minimally differentiated acute leukemia. Leuk Res 1993;17:189–208.

Catovsky D, Matutes E, Buccheri V, et al. A classification of acute leukemia for the 1990s. Ann Hematol 1991;62:16–21.

Cerezo L, Shuster JJ, Pullen DJ, et al. Laboratory correlates and prognostic significance of granular acute lymphoblastic leukemia in children: a Pediatric Oncology Group Study. Am J Clin Path 1991;95:526–531.

Cheson BD, Cassileth PA, Head D, et al. Report of the National Cancer Institute sponsored workshop on definitions of diagnosis and response in acute myeloid leukemia. J Clin Oncol 1990;8:813–819.

Downing JR, Head DR, Raimondi SC, et al. The der(11)-encoded MLL/AF-4 fusion transcript is consistently detected in t(4;11) (q21;q23)-containing acute lymphoblastic leukemia. Blood 1994;83:330–335.

Drexler HG, Borkhardt A, Janssen JW. Detection of chromosomal translocations in leukemia-lymphoma cells by polymerase chain reaction. Leuk Lymphoma 1995;19:359–380.

Dunphy CH, Kitchen S, Sarovia O, et al. Acute myelofibrosis terminating in acute lymphoblastic leukemia: case report and review of the literature. Am J Hematol 1996;51:85–89.

Fauci AS, Harley JB, Roberts WC, et al. The idiopathic hypereosinophilic syndrome: clinical, pathophysiologic, and therapeutic considerations. Ann Intern Med 1982;97:78–92.

Ferrara F, DelVecchio L. Clinical relevance of acute mixed-lineage leukemias. Leuk Lymphoma 1993;12:11–19.

Grigg AP, Gascoyne RD, Phillips GL, et al. Clinical, haematological and cytogenetic features in 24 patients with structural rearrangements of the Q arm of chromosome 3. Br J Haematol 1993;83:158–165.

Hogan TF, Kass W, Murgo AJ, et al. Acute lymphoblastic leukemia with chromosomal 5; 14 translocation and hypereosinophilia: case report and literature review. J Clin Oncol 1987;5:382–390.

Howe RB, Bloomfield CD, McKenna RW. Hypocellular acute leukemia. Am J Med 1982;72:391–395.

Imamura N, Kusunoki Y, Keisi KH, et al. Aggressive natural killer cell leukaemia/lymphoma: report of four cases and review of the literature. Br J Haematol 1990;75:49–59.

Kowal-Vern A, Cotelingam J, Schumacher HR. The prognostic significance of proerythroblasts in acute erythroleukemia. Am J Clin Path 1992;98:34–40.

Lee EJ, Pollak A, Leavitt RD, et al. Minimally differentiated acute nonlymphocytic leukemia: a distinct entity. Blood 1987;70:1400–1406.

Lee M, Chubachi M, Niitsu H, et al. Successful hematopoietic reconstitution with granulocyte-colony-stimulating factor in a patient with hypoplastic acute myelogenous leukemia. Intern Med 1995;34:692–694.

Liang R, Chan TK, Todd D. Childhood acute lymphoblastic leukaemia and aplastic anaemia. Leuk Lymphoma 1994;13:411–415.

Lilleyman JS, Mann IM, Stevens RF, et al. Cytomorphology of childhood lymphoblastic leukemia: a prospective study of 2000 patients. Br J Haematol 1992;81:52–57.

Lillington DM, McCallum TK, Lister TA, et al. Translocation t(6;9)(p23;q34) in acute myeloid leukemia without myelodysplasia or basophilia: two cases and a review of the literature. Leukemia 1993;7:527–531.

Liso V, Specchia G, Pavone V, et al. Acute lymphoblastic leukemia hand mirror cells. Study of nine cases. Blutalkohol 1983;47:297–306.

Loughran TP Jr. Clonal diseases of large granular lymphocytes. Blood 1993;82:1–14.

Matloub YH, Brunning RD, Arther DC, et al. Severe aplastic anemia preceding acute lymphoblastic leukemia. Cancer 1993;71:264–268.

Mazur EM, Wittels EG, Schiffman FJ, et al. Hand mirror lymphoid leukemia in adults: a distinct clinicopathologic syndrome. Case report and literature review. Cancer 1986;57:92–99.

Okamura S, Ikematsu W. Hematological malignancies with eosinophilia. Nippon Rinsho 1993;51(3):800–805.

Peterson LC, Parkin JL, Arthur DC, et al. Acute basophilic leukemia. A clinical, morphologic and cytogenetic study of eight cases. Am J Clin Pathol 1991;96:160–170.

Pui CH. Acute leukemias with t(4;11)(q21;q23). Leuk Lymphoma 1992;7:173–179.

Schoch C, Rieder H, Freund M, et al. Twenty-three cases of acute lymphoblastic leukemia with translocation t(4;11) (q21;q23): the implication of additional chromosomal aberrations. Ann Hematol 1995;70:195–201.

Schumacher HR, Cotelingam JD. Chronic leukemia: approach to diagnosis. New York: Igaku-Shoin, 1993:25–26.

Schumacher HR, Nand S. Myelodysplastic syndromes: approach to diagnosis and treatment. New York: Igaku-Shoin, 1995.

Scott AA, Head DR, Kopecky KJ, et al. HLA-DR-, CD33+, CD56+, CD16-myeloid/natural killer cell acute leukemia: a previously unrecognized form of acute leukemia potentially misdiagnosed as French-American-British acute myeloid leukemia—M3. Blood 1994;84:244–255.

Takizawa J, Kishi K, Moriyama Y, et al. Allogenic bone marrow transplantation for Fanconi's anemia with leukemic transformation from an HLA identical father. Rinsho Ketsueki 1995;36(6):615–620.

Taylor CG, Stasi R, Bastianelli C, et al. Diagnosis and classification of the acute leukemias: recent advances and controversial issues. Hematopathol Mol Hematol 1996;10:1–38.

Venditti A, Del Poeta G, Stasi R, et al. Minimally differentiated acute myeloid leukemia (AML M0): cytochemical, immunophenotypic and cytogenetic analysis of 19 cases. Br J Haematol 1994;88:784–793.

Wegelius R. Preleukaemic states in children. Scand J Haematol Suppl 1986;45:133–139.

Wibowo A, Pankowsky D, Mikhael A, et al. Adult acute leukemia: hand mirror cell variant. Hematopathol Mol Hematol 1996;10:85–98.

Young NS, Maciejewski J. The pathophysiology of acquired aplastic anemia. N Eng J Med 1997;336:1365–1372.

CHAPTER 2

Cytochemistry and Terminal Deoxynucleotidyl Transferase

GENERAL COMMENTS

Morphology and cytochemistry continue to be cornerstones for the diagnosis of acute leukemia. The cytochemical characteristics of the acute lymphoblastic leukemias (ALL) are listed in Table 2.1. Lymphoblasts are negative for myeloperoxidase (MPEX) and chloroacetate esterase (CAE), but very fine positive cytoplasmic granules may be rarely present with Sudan black B (SBB), especially in pediatric ALL. Characteristic block positivity (rosary bead pattern) usually on a clear background with periodic acid-Schiff (PAS) staining may corroborate a diagnosis of ALL, but a similar reactivity may also be observed in AML M6.

Terminal deoxynucleotidyl transferase (TdT) is positive in more than 90% of ALLs; however, it is also positive in some AMLs. Since it is predominately positive in ALLs and in some AMLs, it has been referred to as a lineage-associated marker. An important finding that should be considered to avoid the erroneous diagnosis of ALL is the increase of hematogones in the bone marrow of young children, adolescents, and adults. These are found in bone marrow smears in large numbers in normal infants and older children with nondeficiency, congenital red cell aplasia, neuroblastoma, retinoblastoma, congenital neutropenia, and idiopathic thrombocytopenic purpura. Hematogones may have morphologic features in common with the lymphoblasts of ALL or lymphoblastic lymphoma. Unfortunately, no detailed cytochemical studies have been performed on hematogones. Immunophenotypic analysis of these cells, however, demonstrates a spectrum extending from early B-cell precursors (CD10+, CD19+, TdT+, HLA-DR+) to mature B cells expressing surface immunoglobulins. Specialized techniques, including DNA content analysis, cytogenetics, and molecular analysis, are all normal in bone marrow samples; even when hematogones account for more than 50% of nucleated cells.

Recognition and classification of AML is usually straightforward in the acute leukemias with signs of granulocytic (AML M2 to M4), and monocytic maturation (AML M5b). The AML M2, M3, and M4 demonstrate a variable percentage of blasts with type II features (up to 21 granules). Those cases classified as AML M1 and M5a contain type I blasts (absent granules) and are more dependent on cytochemical stains.

The AML M6 is discussed later in this chapter and presented in Case 4 in Chapter 8. The MPEX and PAS are important stains in the diagnosis. Many of those cases associated with the presence of myeloblasts represent an evo-

Table 2.1
Cytochemistries of the Acute Lymphoblastic Leukemias

FAB Type	MPEX	SBB	AP^a	A-EST	B-EST	CAE	C-EST A-EST	C-EST CAE	PAS	Iron	MGP	ORO	TdT	Comment
L1	−	− (rare+)	+	+ (weak)	− (weak focal)	−	+ (weak)	−	+/− (block)	−	+	− (rare+)	+	Small lymphoid elements. Bead necklace PAS+
L2	−	− (rare+)	+	+ (weak)	− (weak focal)	−	+ (weak)	−	+/− (block)	−	+	− (rare+)	+	Large heterogeneous lymphoblasts. Confused with M1, M4, M5
L3	−	−	+	−	−	−	−	−	− (rare+)	−	+ (strong)	+ (vacuoles)	− (very rare+)	Large homogeneous lymphoblasts. Deep basophilic vacuolated cytoplasm. PAS-, Tdt-, ORO+ MGP strongly+

^a Focal unipolar positivity—T-ALL (see abbreviations).

lution of a previous myelodysplastic syndrome. In order to establish the diagnosis of AML M0 and AML M7, light cytochemical stains are not sufficient. Additional immunologic and/or ultrastructural studies are always necessary. Ultrastructural studies on AML M0 demonstrate MPEX reactivity that may be present in the granules, nuclear envelope, and endoplasmic reticulum. Similar studies in AML M7 to show platelet peroxidase (PPO) have been employed; however, the PPO is characteristically only present in the perinuclear cistern and endoplasmic reticulum, but not in the Golgi region or small granules. The FAB classification with the cytochemical reaction of the various AMLs is presented in Table 2.2.

ACUTE UNDIFFERENTIATED LEUKEMIA (AUL)

These cases are undefined by morphological, cytochemical, immunological, and ultrastructural analysis. They account for only 1 to 3% of the acute leukemias and continue to decrease as biotechnology enables us to assign lineage to such cases. Receptor studies, gene expression, and in vitro culture studies may, in the near future, contribute substantially to our knowledge about the commitment of these undifferentiated or minimally differentiated blasts. In this regard, Crisan and Anstett have analyzed seven cases with morphology and cytochemistry consistent with AUL. They utilized a procedure for MPEX messenger ribonucleic acid (mRNA) detection by RT-PCR that was adopted for use on routine hematology smears. MPEX mRNA was detected in six of the seven cases establishing the myeloid lineage of the blasts and the diagnosis of AML M0. In the remaining case, the blasts were MPEX mRNA-negative, confirming a diagnosis of AUL (Table 2.3).

ACUTE LYMPHOBLASTIC LEUKEMIA (ALL)

Hypocellular/Aplastic Acute Leukemia

Reports of cytochemical stains on aplastic/hypocellular ALL are sparse in the literature. Empirically, one would expect that they stain similar to other ALLs. Hatta et al. reported a complete remission induced by granulocyte-colony-stimulating factor (G-CSF) in a patient with hypoplastic ALL that demonstrated myeloperoxidase negative and CD2- and CD7-positive markers in a T-ALL.

Granular ALL

Although granular ALL is relatively infrequent; cytochemical stains can generally facilitate in the distinction of it from myelogenous leukemias. The constant positivity of the granules for acid phosphatase and/or nonspecific esterase strongly suggests their lysosomal origin. In addition, the granules are MPEX and CAE negative, but approximately 20% of the cases will exhibit SBB positivity. PAS has been reported to be weakly positive in some cases. Some cases have coexpressed myeloid antigens and others have

Table 2.2
Cytochemistries of the Acute Myeloid Leukemias[a]

FAB Type	MPEX	SBB	AP	A-EST	B-EST	CAE	C-EST		PAS	Iron	MGP	ORO	TdT	Comment
							A-EST	CAE						
M0	−	−	+	−	−	−	−	−	+/−	−	+/−	−	+/−	≥20% blasts express one or more antigens: CD13, CD14, CD33. Negative for lymphoid antigens (exception: CD7 and TdT may be +)
M1	+	+	+	+/− (weak)	−	+/−	+/− (weak)	+/−	+/−	−	+/−	−	−/+	>90% myeloblasts, MPEX+, B-EST−
[b]M2	+	+	+	+/− (weak)	−	+/−	+/− (weak)	+/−	+/−	−	+/−	−	−/+	>10% granulocytic cells. Auer rods common
[c]M3	+	+	+	+/− (weak)	−	+/−	+/− (weak)	+/−	+/−	−	+/−	−	−/+	Numerous promyelocytes. Faggot cells common
[b]M4	+	+	+	+ (NaF-S)[d]	+	+/− (NaF-S)	+ (NaF-S)	+ (NaF-S)	+/−	−	+/−	−	−/+	Myelocytic and monocytic series present. Lineage infidelity. Monocytic series NaF-S
[e]M5	+/−	+/−	+	+ (NaF-S)	+	+/− (NaF-S)	+/− (NaF-S)	+/− (NaF-S)	+/−	−	+/−	−	−/+	Clefted cells present usually. B-EST+, A-EST+, NaF-S
M6A	+	+	+	+/− (weak)	−	+/−	+/− (weak)	+/−	+/− (Diffuse and block)	+/− (Ringed sideroblasts)	+/−	−	−/+	Myeloblasts predominate (DiGuglielmo's syndrome)
M6B	−	−	+	+/− (weak)	−	−	+/− (weak)	−	+/− (Diffuse and block)	+/− (Ringed sideroblasts)	+	−	−	Proerythroblasts predominate (DiGuglielmo's disease)
M7	−	−	+	+ (NaF-S)	−	−	+ (NaF-S)	−	+ (Coarse granules)	−	+/−	−	−	Sometimes peripheral blood diagnosis. Immunopheno-type and EM platelet peroxidase can be **diagnostic**

[a] See abbreviations for stains.
[b] M2 EO, M4 EO—Eosinophils stain abnormally PAS, CAE positive.
[c] M3v—microgranules variant stains similarly. EM helpful to show granules.
[d] NaF-S—sodium fluoride sensitive.
[e] M5a—undifferentiated MPEX, SBB usually negative. M5b—differentiated MPEX, SBB may be positive.

demonstrated myeloperoxidase by transmission electron microscopy. Such findings suggest phenotypic variation, which is supported by the finding that a higher incidence of azurophilic granules are present in those ALLs that co-express myeloid antigens.

ALL with Eosinophilia

Contrary to the abnormal eosinophils of the myelogenous leukemias, the eosinophils of lymphoid malignancies result because of stimulating cytokines, including IL3, IL5, and granulocyte-macrophage colony-stimulating factor (GM-CSF). These eosinophils are normal and demonstrate strong reactivity with MPEX, SBB, and moderate reactivity with naphthol-AS and α-naphthyl esterase. They do not show activity with toluidine blue, alkaline phosphatase, CAE, Astra blue, or PAS.

The observation of CAE and PAS activity in some abnormal eosinophils is of particular interest in view of the subsequent finding that abnormal eosinophils in acute myelomonocytic leukemia are associated with inversion of chromosome 16. Most of the patients studied had a higher than normal percentage of immature abnormal eosinophils, containing a mixture of eosinophilic and basophilic granules (Fig. 2.1). Normally, the eosinophilic and basophilic granules are mutually exclusive in respect to granulocytic lineage; however, the presence of both granules in CML cells is a sign of lineage infidelity.

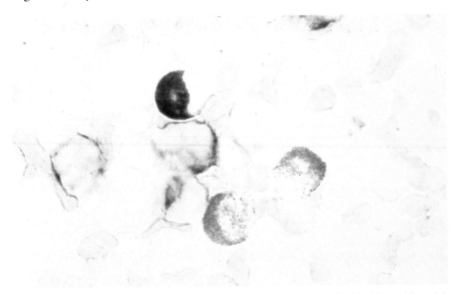

Figure 2.1. Bone marrow from a patient with FAB AML M4Eo stained with chlorazol fast pink for eosinophils (red), and CAE fast blue RR for other granulocytic elements (blue). Note dark staining cell with both red and blue stain (abnormal eosinophil). This confirms abnormal eosinophils in FAB AML M4Eo stain with CAE (×1000). Courtesy of James Vardiman.

Table 2.3
Summary of Cytochemistry and TdT

Diagnosis FAB Subtype	Cytochemistry	Comment	References
AUL	Undefined by cyto-chemistry	Fewer of these cases will be reported as biotech-nology advances. MPEX mRNA can be detected by RT-PCR	Leukemia 1990;4:620–624
Hypocellular/ aplastic ALL	Sparse reports in litera-ture. Would expect cases to stain similar to other ALLs	Rare report of complete remission with G-CSF	Haematologica 1995;94:39–43
Granular ALL	Granules acid phos-phatase and/or nonspecific esterase positive. MPEX, CAE negative, but 20% SBB positive	Some cases have co-ex-pressed myeloid anti-gens and demonstrated MPEX by EM. Findings suggest phenotypic variation which is sup-ported by higher inci-dence of azurophilic granules in ALLs that co-express myeloid antigens	Am J Clin Pathol 1983;79:426–430
ALL with eosinophilia	Eosinophils strongly posi-tive for MPEX, SBB. Moderate reactivity with naphthol-AS, A-EST. PAS, CAE, Astra blue, toluidine blue negative.	Eosinophils reactive from stimulation by cy-tokines from tumor. Do not stain positive with PAS and CAE	Acta Haematologica 1993;90:144–147
Acute leukemia with t(4;11)	MPEX and SBB may be present in some cases. NSE may be positive in variable number of cells	High frequency of mixed lineage in ALL cases exhibiting either t(4;11) or t(9;22)	Blood 1986;67:689–697
Acute leukemia Hand mirror variant (ALL-HMV)	Variable depending on HMV reported. Initial ALL,−HMV PAS+, AP+, TdT+. FAB M4, M5 HMV − MPEX+, SBB+, B-EST+, A-EST+, C-EST+	Mixed lineage cases have demonstrated variable staining patterns. Im-munophenotyping sup-ported mixed lineage	Hematopathol Mol Hematol 1996; 10:85–86
Aggressive natural killer cell leukemia (ANKCL)	Usually AP (tartrate sen-sitive) +, B-EST+, B-glucuronidase+. MPEX−, CAE−, PAS−, LAP−	May be mistaken for neuroblastoma	Br J Haematol 1990;75:49–59

Table 2.3   *(Continued)*

Diagnosis FAB Subtype	Cytochemistry	Comment	References
AML-M0	Blasts <3% positive for SBB/MPEX, TdT may be positive	Diagnosis established by immunophenotyping and/or EM-MPEX	Blood 1997;89:621–629
AML M6A, M6B Erythroleukemia	M6A MPEX positive myeloblasts. M6B MPEX negative in proerythroblasts. Both groups show PAS blush and block positivity in erythroid cell line. Ringed sideeroblasts present in both.	Important to separate into M6A and M6B, since survival is much better in M6A	Am J Clin Pathol 1992; 98:526–530
Acute basophilic leukemia (ABL)	Usually negative for MPEX, SBB. Toluidine blue, astra blue, Giemsa positive for basophilic granules. Blasts may be negative	EM may be necessary to establish diagnosis	Cancer 1995;75: 110–114
Eosinophilic leukemia (EL) Hypereosino-philic syn-drome (HES)	PAS, CAE positive granules in EL eosinophils	Normal eosinophils may demonstrate positive intergranular (cytoplasmic) staining	Br J Haematol 1987; 67:25–31
Hypocellular AML	Variable depending FAB subtype M0 MPEX−, SBB− M1 MPEX+, SBB+ M2 MPEX+, SBB+	Rare cases of M6 and M7 reported	Leukemia Res 1996; 20:563–574 Hematol Pathol 1995;9:195–203
CD7 positive AML	Cases predominately M0, M1, M5a. Cytochemistries correlate with FAB subtype	Controversy over prognosis and clinical findings in these cases may be related to antibodies to CD7.	Am J Clin Pathol 1996; 106:185–191
AML 3(q21;q26)	Cases predominately M1, M4, M6. Cytochemistries correlate with FAB subtype	Abnormalities in megakaryocytopoiesis. Normal platelet counts or thrombocytosis	Blood 1985;66:1362–1370
Myeloid/NK leukemia	MPEX+, SBB+, CAE+, PAS weakly+/−	Confused with M3. t(15;17) negative. Fails to respond to ATRA	Blood 1994;84:244–255
Biphenotypic bilineage acute leukemia	Not of great use. Most schemes dependent on immunophenotypic markers. Biphenotypics show low percentage of MPEX+ blasts. Bilineal usually stain appropriately for each lineage	Controversial area where no strict criteria are of value. Matutes, Catovsky scoring system used at University of Cincinnati Medical Center	Leuk Lymphoma 13: 1994;1(Suppl):11–14

ALL t(4;11)

There is a much higher frequency of selected mixed lineage in ALL cases exhibiting either t(4;11) (often CD15 coexpression) or t(9;22) (usually CD13 or CD33 coexpression) karyotypes. Besides myeloid antigen expression, some of these cases exhibit other myeloid features such as cytoplasmic granules or expression of G-CSF receptors. For this reason, positive staining for MPEX or SBB may be present in some cases; and the nonspecific esterase reaction may be positive in a variable number of cells. Patients with the t(4;11) have a unique immunophenotype in virtually all cases, the blasts are CD19+/CD10−, HLA-DR+ and TdT+. Although TdT is positive in over 90% of ALLs, it may also be positive in a small percentage of AMLs. Therefore, it is lineage associated, but not lineage specific.

ALL-Hand Mirror Variant (ALL-HMV)

The results of cytochemical staining of various cases reported in the literature varied with the classification of the HMV. In the initial group reported by Mazur et al., the patients had ALL-HMV. They showed female predominance, a relatively indolent early course, failure to achieve a complete remission with chemotherapy and Ia-positive null cells. Cytochemical staining revealed PAS+, acid phosphatase+, myeloperoxidase−, SBB−, non-specific esterases—hand mirror cells (HMVs). The PAS stain of the HMV demonstrated coarse granules and block positivity. In some cells, coarse granules formed a necklace around the nucleus and extended into the uropod (Fig. 2.2). In others, the stain was concentrated in the uropod. The area between the granules and blocks of PAS-positive material was usually clear and did not show the diffuse background stain noted in myeloid leukemias. The acid phosphatase stain was granular and concentrated mainly in the uropod in those cells that formed hand mirrors (Fig. 2.3). The acid phosphatase stain was inhibited by tartrate in this group of ALL-HMV patients. TdT was positive over the nucleus, which may extend into the uropod. In addition to ALL-HMV, Haider et al. reported three HMVs that were myeloid. Two were classified as FAB M4 and one was FAB M5. The FAB M5 was butyrate esterase and SBB+. The two FAB M4 cases showed both myelocytic and monocytic morphology and were positive for MPEX, SBB, B-EST, A-EST, and C-EST.

Recently, Kovarik et al. reported an ALL-HMV that demonstrated a mixed immunophenotype. The blast cells were found to be pre B cells (CD19+ and TdT+) that also expressed myeloid antigens (CD13, CD33) and demonstrated a heavy chain immunoglobulin gene rearrangement. Cytogenetic studies revealed a t(11;19) previously described in biphenotypic leukemias. Cytochemical stains revealed positive PAS with a perinuclear "rosary bead" pattern in the HMCs. Acid phosphatase stain demonstrated diffuse positivity in the HMCs, while the myeloperoxidase and SBB stains were negative.

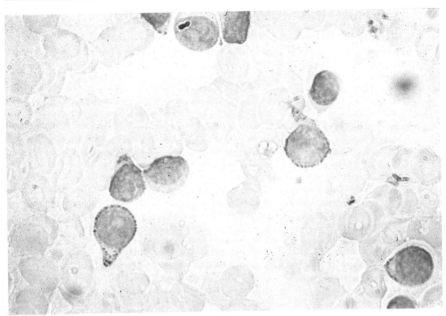

Figure 2.2. Bone marrow from patient with ALL-HMV. PAS reaction shows rosary bead pattern and large granules in the tip of the uropod in hand mirror cell (upper left) (×1000).

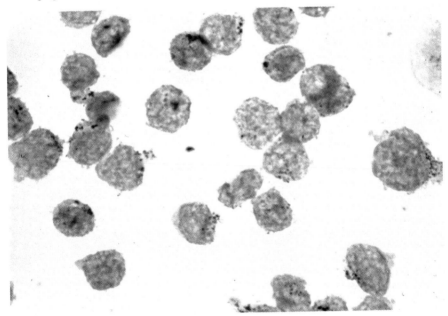

Figure 2.3. Bone marrow from a patient with ALL-HMV stained for acid phosphatase. Note granular punctate positivity. Also, note lack of numerous hand mirror cells due to crowded cellular area (×1000).

More recently, Wibowo et al. reported two cases of acute mixed HMV leukemia with strong expression of CD2, CD7, and CD11b that were myeloperoxidase +, SBB+, alpha-naphthyl acetate esterase +, and TdT+. The authors emphasized the importance of the adhesion molecule CD2. Such molecules on activated HMCs is important to homing, trafficking, spread of malignant cells, clinical course, prognosis, and treatment.

Aggressive NK Cell Leukemia (ANKCL)

This aggressive disorder is characterized by a phenotype that is CD3−, CD8−, and CD56+. These cases represent a minority of those cases with medium- to large-granulated lymphocytes. In ANKCL, the cells are usually large and undifferentiated, demonstrate prominent nucleoli, and have a moderate amount of basophilic cytoplasm, which has been vacuolated in rare cases. These cells usually show reactivity for beta-glucuronidase and tartrate-sensitive acid phosphatase. Imamura et al. reported four cases and reviewed seven cases of ANKCL from the literature. Over 80% of lymphoid cells from patients were positive for acid phosphatase (tartrate sensitive), α-naphthyl butyrate esterase, and B-glucuronidase (Fig. 2.4). They were neg-

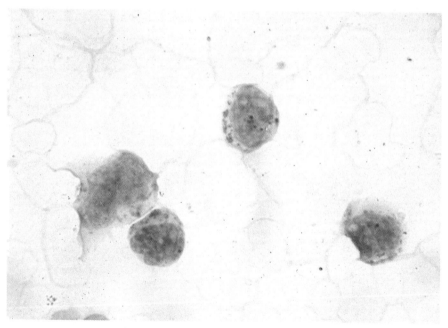

A

Figure 2.4. A. Peripheral blood showing acid phosphatase positive NK cells. Note large granular positivity (×1000). Courtesy of Nobutaka Imamura. B. Bone marrow demonstrating B-EST positive NK cells. Stain diffusely involves cytoplasm of NK cells (×1000). Courtesy of Nobutaka Imamura. C. Bone marrow exhibiting B-glucuronidase positive NK cells. Stain is cytoplasmic, diffuse, and finely granular (×1000). Courtesy of Nobutaka Imamura.

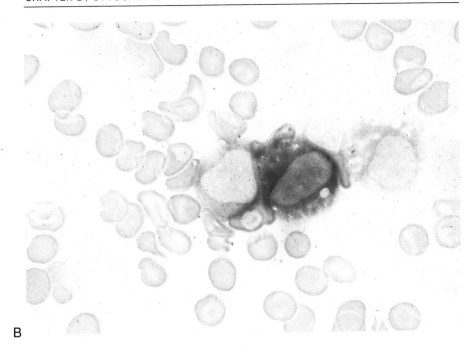

B

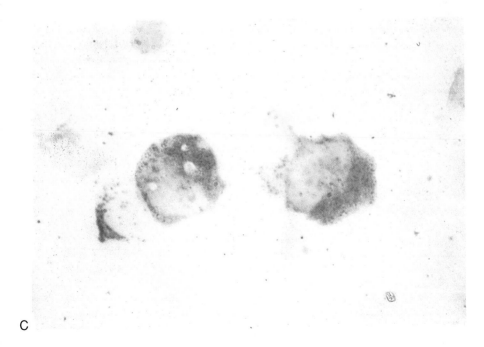

C

ative for MPEX, CAE, PAS, and leukocyte alkaline phosphatase. Gardiner et al. reported a case that initially was diagnosed as neuroblastoma. Cyto-chemistry was noncontributory since the malignant cells were negative for myeloperoxidase, SBB, PAS, TdT, and esterase stains. Brody et al. reported a case in which PAS+ vacuoles were observed. The abnormal cells showed focal tartrate-sensitive positivity. This case was unusual in that the cells were agranular, CD4+, and CD56+. Both of the above cases only survived for approximately 6 months.

ACUTE MYELOID LEUKEMIA (AML)

AML M0

A case is defined as AML M0 when the minimally differentiated blast cells are SBB/MPEX negative or less than 3% positive. The lymphoid markers are negative, with the exception of CD7 and TdT, which may be positive. If 20% or more blasts express one or more myeloid antigens (CD13, CD14, CD33), a diagnosis of AML M0 can be established. Monoclonal antibody to MPEX may be more sensitive than cytochemical MPEX (Fig. 2.5). Also, if ultrastructural MPEX is positive, a diagnosis is confirmed. The MPEX re-activity may be present in the granules, the nuclear envelope, and the endo-

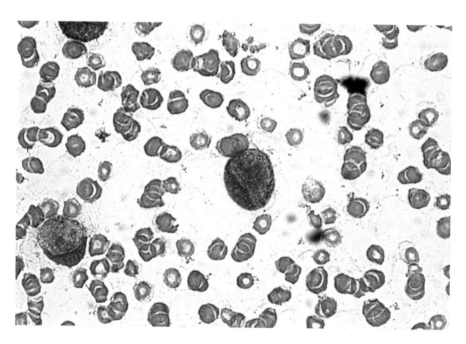

Figure 2.5. Bone marrow from patient with FAB AML M0 stained with myeloid-specific anti-bodies to MPEX by alkaline phosphatase anti-alkaline phosphatase technique. Note diffuse pos-itive reddish brown stain in the cytoplasm (×1000). Courtesy of Roberto Stasi.

plasmic reticulum. In AML M0 the number of cells reactive with MPEX by EM varies, but is usually less than 50% of the blasts.

AML M6-Erythroleukemia

The classification of this disorder is dependent on cytochemical stains. FAB M6 only considers Di Guglielmo's syndrome, which contains significant numbers of myeloblasts; however, there is another form of erythroleukemia that is referred to as Di Guglielmo's disease or pure erythroleukemia. We designate the syndrome M6A and the disease M6B.

Kowal-Vern et al. studied cytochemical stains and TdT on 23 cases of erythroleukemia (10 M6A, 13 M6B). All 10 patients with M6A had positive MPEX staining of myeloblasts, whereas only 1 of 13 M6B patients had positivity in rare myeloblasts. Twelve of thirteen M6B cases (93%) and six of eight M6A cases (75%) had PAS block and granular positivity in the proerythroblasts and erythroid precursors. The A-EST was positive in the blasts of six of eight (75%) in M6A, but only in two of seven M6B cases (29%). The C-EST stain was positive in six of seven M6A cases (86%) and in three of five M6B cases (60%). The CAE stained the more mature granulocytic elements in both groups. The A-EST portion of the C-EST correlated with the findings of the A-EST alone. Iron stores varied from 2 to 4+ in both groups. Ringed sideroblasts were present in 18 of 23 patients (86%). The five patients who did not have ringed sideroblasts had a high percentage of very immature erythroblasts and belonged predominately to the M6B group. TdT was performed by indirect immunofluorescence on a total of 10 patients from both groups and was consistently negative.

Cytochemical stains on M6 are demonstrated in Figures 2.6A and B.

Acute Basophilic Leukemia (ABL)

Basophilic leukemia is a rare heterogeneous disorder that has been associated with AMLs with t(6;9), t(3;6), and inv (16) chromosomal abnormalities. Also, cases of acute promyelocytic leukemia with basophilic maturation have been reported. In addition, de novo acute basophilic leukemia exists and may demonstrate symptoms related to histamine release and disseminated intravascular coagulation.

Besides acute situations, basophilic leukemia may occur in the chronic phase of CML or as a manifestation of the accelerated phase of CML (Fig. 2.7). Finally, it may present a Ph[1] negative LAP positive de novo chronic leukemia. Such cases need to be evaluated for bcr rearrangement.

The basophilic circulating cells and blasts are usually negative for MPEX and SBB stains. However, the SBB reaction may show a peculiar reddish metachromatic hue with only occasional block granules in abnormal basophils, even when the granules are inconspicuous. Although the toluidine blue, Astra blue, and Giemsa stains are frequently reactive with basophilic

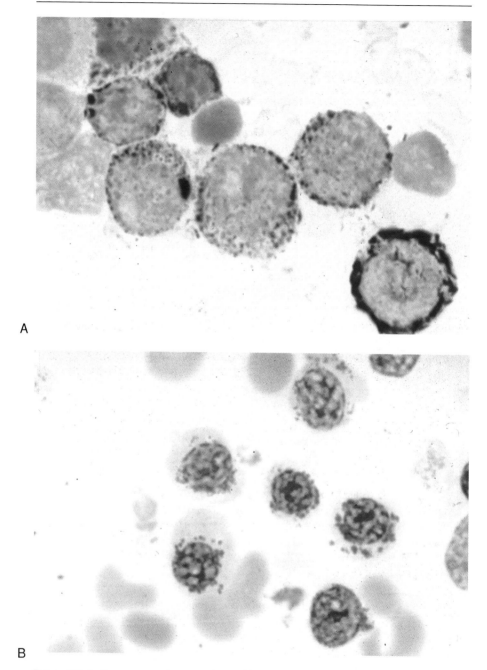

A

B

Figure 2.6. A. Bone marrow from a patient with acute erythroleukemia (M6B), Di Guglielmo's disease. PAS reaction exhibiting blush granular and block positivity in erythroid precursors (×1000). B. Note numerous ringed sideroblasts. Acute erythroleukemia (M6B), BM (×1000).

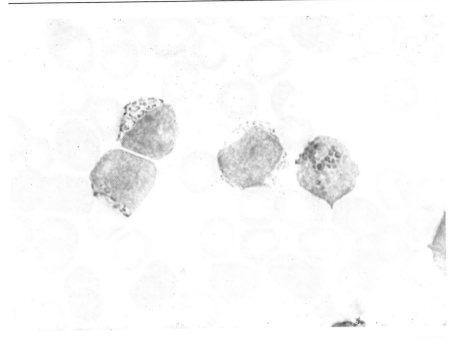

Figure 2.7. Peripheral blood showing toluidine blue positive basophilic blasts in a case of CML in basophilic blast crisis. Positive granules are large and extend over the nucleus on blast on right (×1000). Courtesy of Daniel Pankowsky.

granules, blast cells may be negative. Such cases may make the diagnosis extremely difficult and require additional diagnostic studies, including transmission electron microscopy (Fig. 2.8). Amino caproate esterase staining reaction has been used by some investigators to identify mast cells. It is sensitive to storage and heat, and the incubation is unduly prolonged; therefore, it has not gained wide popularity. The PAS reaction in basophils at all stages of maturity may be increased in CML and myeloproliferative disorders, with coarse granularity and block-type positivity. PAS may also be positive in mast cells.

Eosinophilic Leukemia (EL)/Hypereosinophilic Syndrome (HES)

Early in the course of eosinophilic leukemia (EL) and hypereosinophilic syndrome (HES), it is usually impossible to establish a diagnosis. Both diseases usually reveal leukocyte counts well over 20×10^9/L and absolute eosinophil counts of greater than 1.5×10^9/L sustained for at least 6 months. The characterization of a hypereosinophilic process as leukemia has traditionally been based on the presence of immature cells in the blood or blast transformation. Although blast transformation should be considered evidence for leukemia, the presence of immature cells of the granulocytic series in the blood is not in itself sufficient for a diagnosis of leukemia. Such

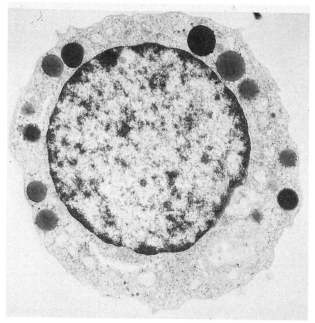

Figure 2.8. Electron micrograph of basophilic blast from same case as in Figure 2.6. Nucleus only contains small amount of heterochromatin; granules appear homogeneous, but at higher magnification are finely particulate (×6000). No theta granules were found even after a diligent search. Courtesy of Daniel Pankowsky.

cases should be evaluated by cytogenetic analysis to determine the presence of a clonal chromosomal abnormality that would support a diagnosis of leukemia.

In addition to morphological abnormalities of nuclear-cytoplasmic dyssynchrony, hypersegmentation and hyposegmentation of nuclei, enlarged secondary granules, pronounced hypogranularity of the cytoplasm, and cytoplasmic vacuoles, two cytochemical reactions, PAS and CAE, have been used to distinguish benign from malignant eosinophils. In EL, the abnormal granules stain positive with CAE and PAS; whereas, normal eosinophilic granules are negative for these stains. Nevertheless, it is important to note that normal eosinophils may demonstrate PAS-positive intergranular (cytoplasmic) staining. MPEX usually stains both leukemic and normal eosinophils in a similar manner. A recent report by Aldebert et al. has provided evidence that human eosinophils express a functional receptor for alpha interferon. Such a finding represents a potential basis for the beneficial effects of alpha interferon in patients with hypereosinophilic syndromes. Additional information on eosinophilic leukemia can be found in Case 2 in Chapter 8.

Hypocellular AML

Hypocellular AML is defined as a condition with 30% or more blasts in bone marrow that is less than 30% cellular, as based on an adequate biopsy. Since hypocellular AML occurs predominately in patients 50 years or older, frequently evolving from an MDS, some authors have used less than 20% cellularity in older patients. This diagnosis does not imply a specific FAB diagnosis, however, the majority of cases are AML M0, AML M1, or AML M2. Yamato et al. reported a case of severe aplastic anemia that evolved into a FAB M6. In addition, cases of hypocellular AML may occur in infants with AML M7. As discussed previously, the differential diagnosis of hypocellular AML can be extremely difficult, and includes aplastic anemia and hypocellular MDS.

The cytochemical stains of these various hypocellular leukemias will vary. In the FAB M0 less than 3% of the blasts are positive for MPEX, SBE, or nonspecific esterase, whereas, $\geq$ 20% blasts express one or more myeloid antigens: CD13, CD14, CD33, or ultrastructural peroxidase. FAB M1 and M2 stain with MPEX and SBB. PAS stain usually demonstrates a diffuse pink tinge with or without evidence of superimposed granules. On the contrary, the PAS stain in the lymphoblastic leukemias show a necklace of coarse granules on a clear background. FAB M6 stains a population of myeloblasts with MPEX and SBB. Remember, the pure erythroleukemia (M6B) is negative for MPEX and SBB since almost all the leukemic cells are erythroid precursors. PAS stains the erythroid cells in a block (usually proerythroblasts) and blush (usually more mature erythroid elements) manner. Ringed sideroblasts are common (Case 4, Chapter 8). The megakaryoblasts of FAB M7 are MPEX and SBB negative. They are B-EST negative and are A-EST positive-fluoride sensitive. The latter being presumptive evidence for a diagnosis of FAB M7. The acid phosphatase reaction may be positive, with scattered granules displayed in a nonspecific pattern. Since FAB M7 may be diagnosed by immunophenotypic analysis, a number of monoclonal antibodies to platelet glycoproteins have been utilized. They include CD41, directed against platelet gp IIb/IIIa, CD42b directed against platelet gp Ib, and CD61 directed against platelet gp IIIa. Antibodies to factor VIII-related antigen are less sensitive in the identification of megakaryoblasts. Ultrastructural platelet peroxidase may be necessary to establish the diagnosis in some cases. Characteristically, the platelet peroxidase reaction product is deposited in the perinuclear cistern and endoplasmic reticulum, but not in the Golgi region or small granules.

CD7-Positive AML

CD7 is expressed in 10% to 30% of AML cases: most frequently in FAB M0, M1, M5a and in association with immature markers such as CD34, TdT, and HLA-DR. Venditti studied 200 consecutive cases of AML and identified 19 cases of FAB M0. Cytochemistry including MPEX, SBB, A-EST, B-EST, CAE, AP, and PAS were negative in 14 cases, 5 cases expressing a very faint cytoplasmic B-EST, and A-EST, which was fluoride sensitive. CD7 was positive in six cases and TdT was expressed in nine. All the cases were antiMPEX positive and phenotypic analysis revealed myeloid features, with all the patients displaying at least one myeloid antigen (CD13, CD33, CD15). FAB M1 would be positive for MPEX and SBB; however, CAE is not present until the promyelocyte stage, and, unless blasts with granules are present (type II blasts), the reaction will be negative. The monoblasts of FAB M5a may be MPEX and SBB positive or negative. The blasts are usually A-EST and B-EST positive and both are sensitive to sodium fluoride. In my experience, the B-EST is more specific and less sensitive than the A-EST. The leukemic cells may be CAE positive or negative. If positive, the CAE is sensitive to sodium fluoride. Since cases of FAB M5a with CD7 represent cases with immature markers, cytochemical analysis may be more difficult.

AML inv 3(q21;q26)

These cases of AML have been associated with normal platelet counts or thrombocytosis. They generally have associated abnormalities of megakaryocytopoiesis, including increased megakaryocytes and micromegakaryocytes. AMLs with abnormalities of the long arm of chromosome 3 are difficult to classify morphologically, with cases of FAB M1, M4, and M6 reported in the literature. The FAB M1 cases would be MPEX and SBB positive; the FAB M4 cases MPEX, SBB, B-EST, and C-EST positive. The esterase stains would be partially sensitive to fluoride. The FAB M6 cases may be MPEX and SBB positive or negative. PAS usually is positive, with block positivity in the proerythroblasts and blush positivity in the more mature erythroid precursors. Iron stain frequently reveals ringed sideroblasts.

Myeloid/NK Leukemia

These unusual cases were previously unrecognized and apparently classified as acute promyelocytic leukemia, FAB M3, that did not respond to all-trans-retinoic acid. Multicolor flow cytometric assays confirmed the coexpression of myeloid (CD33, CD13, CD15), and NK cell (CD56) associated antigens in these cases. Such cases lack the t(15;17) and the promyelocytic/retinoic acid receptor alpha fusion transcript by RT-PCR assays. The leukemic blasts in the majority of these cases share unique morphological features (deeply invaginated nuclear membranes and scant cytoplasm with fine azurophilic granularity). These fine granules demonstrate MPEX and SBB positivity that is remarkably similar to those of acute promyelocytic leukemia (FAB AML M3), especially the microgranular variant (FAB AML M3v). CAE should be positive in these cases. Esterase stains should be weak to absent and PAS stain should show a diffuse weak positivity or total absence.

BILINEAGE/BIPHENOTYPIC ACUTE LEUKEMIA

In general, the use of cytochemical staining in these leukemias has not been of great use. Most of the diagnostic schemes have depended heavily on immunophenotypic markers.

In ALLs that express characteristics of more than one lineage, PAS staining may be present in blasts with predominantly lymphoid or myeloid characteristics. Also, even though most PAS-negative cases have predominantly myeloid characteristics, a few have an expression of almost entirely lymphoid-associated characteristics.

Myeloperoxidase has been employed in some diagnostic schemes; however, cases with a high percentage of MPEX-positive blasts rarely meet the criteria of biphenotypic leukemia. The biphenotypic leukemias usually demonstrate a low percentage of MPEX blasts. Although SBB staining is strongly associated with AML, some ALLs have been reported to be positive. Nevertheless, those cases of biphenotypic leukemia studied with MPEX and SBB staining showed concordance.

The B-EST staining is usually negative in biphenotypic leukemia unless the cells show distinct monocytic features. These rare cases usually have been classified as FAB AML M4 or M5 in the past, and must be carefully analyzed to ensure that the binding of monoclonal antibodies is not due to nonspecific Fc antibody binding.

Transmission electron microscopy may reveal lineage characteristics of myeloid or lymphoid differentiation. Both MPEX and PPO can be used to one's advantage to define myeloid and megakaryocytic lineage, respectively.

BIBLIOGRAPHY

Articles

Aldebert D, Lamkhioued B, Desaint C, et al. Eosinophils express a functional receptor for interferon alpha: inhibitory role of interferon alpha on the release of mediators. Blood 1996;87:2354–2360.

Arthur DC, Bloomfield CD, Lindquist LL, et al. Translocation 4;11 in acute lymphoblastic leukemia: clinical characteristics and prognostic significance. Blood 1982;59:96–99.

Bassan R, Biondi A, Benvistito S, et al. Acute undifferentiated leukemia with CD7+ and CD13+ immunophenotype. Lack of molecular lineage commitment and association with poor prognostic features. Cancer 1992;69:396–404.

Brody JP, Allen S, Schulman P, et al. Acute agranular CD4-positive natural killer cell leukemia: comprehensive clinicopathologic studies including virologic and in vitro culture with inducing agents. Cancer 1995;75:2474–2483.

Crisan D, Anstett MJ. Myeloperoxidase mRNA detection for lineage determination of leukemic blasts: retrospective analysis. Leukemia 1995;9:1264–1275.

Davis, RE, Longacre TA, Cornbleet PJ. Hematogones in the bone marrow of adults. Am J Clin Pathol 1994;102:207–211.

Ferrara F, DelVecchio L. Clinical relevance of acute mixed-lineage leukemias. Leuk Lymphoma 1993;12:11–19.

Gardiner CM, Reen DJ, O'Meara A. Recognition of unusual presentation of natural killer cell leukemia. Am J Hematol 1995;50:133–139.

Haider YS, Phillips TM, Schumacher HR. Acute myeloid cells with hand mirror cells. Arch Pathol Lab Med 1982;106:271–274.

Hatta Y, Iwata T, Takeuchi J, et al. Complete remission in a patient with hypoplastic acute lymphoblastic leukemia induced by granulocyte-colony-stimulating factor. Acta Haematologica 1995;94:39–43.

Kovarik P, Shrit MA, Yuen B, et al. Hand mirror variant of adult acute lymphoblastic leukemia: Evidence for a mixed leukemia. Am J Clin Pathol 1992;98:526–530.

Kowal-Vern A, Cotelingam J, Schumacher HR. The prognostic significance of proerythroblasts in acute erythroleukemia. Am J Clin Pathol 1992;98:34–40.

Liso V, Troceoli G, Specchia G, et al. Cytochemical "normal" and "abnormal" eosinophils in acute leukemias. Am J Hematol 1977;2:123–131.

Matutes E, Catovsky D. The value of scoring systems for the diagnosis of biphenotypic leukemia and mature B-cell disorders. Leuk Lymphoma 1994;13(Supp 1):11–14.

Mirro J, Kitchingham G, Williams D, et al. Clinical and laboratory characteristics of acute leukemia with the 4;11 translocation. Blood 1986;67:689–697.

Nagai K, Kohno T, Chen YX, et al. Diagnostic criteria for hypocellular acute leukemia and myelodysplastic syndrome. Leukemia Res 1996;20:563–574.

Ohmoto A, Kohno M, Matsuyama R, et al. Acute lymphocytic leukemia with thrombophlebitis of lower limbs and translocation 4;11. Rinsho Ketsueki 1990;31:l827–1830.

Sandhaus LM, Chen TL, Ettinger LJ, et al. Significance of increased proportion of CD-positive cells in nonmalignant bone marrows of children. Am J Pediatr Hematol Oncol 1993;15:65–70.

Scott AA, Head DR, Kopecky KJ, et al. HLA-DR-CD33+, CD56+, CD16− myeloid/natural killer cell acute leukemia: a previously unrecognized form of acute leukemia potentially misdiagnosed as FAB M3. Blood 1994;84:244–255.

Venditti A, DelPoeta G, Stasi R, et al. Minimally differentiated acute myeloid leukemia (AML-M0): cytochemical, immunophenotypic, and cytogenetic analysis of 19 cases. Br J Haematol 1994;88:784–793.

Venditti A, DelPoeta G, Buccisano F, et al. Minimally differentiated acute myeloid leukemia (AML-M0): comparison of 25 cases with other French-American-British subtypes. Blood 1997;89:621–629.

Review Articles

Catovsky, Matutes E, Buccheri V, et al. A classification of acute leukemia for the 1990s. Ann Hematol 1991;62:16–21.

Foucar K. Acute lymphoblastic leukemia. In: Foucar K. Bone marrow pathology. Chicago: ASCP Press, 1994:382.

Hurwitz CA, Mirro J. Mixed-lineage leukemia and asynchronous antigen expression. Hematol Oncol Clin North Am 1990;4:767–794.

Imamura N, Kusunoki Y, Kawa-Ha K, et al. Aggressive natural killer cell leukaemia/lymphoma: report of four cases and review of literature. Br J Haematol 1990;75:49–59.

Klobusicka M. Possibilities and limitations of cytochemical methods in diagnosis of acute leukemia. Micron 1994;25:317–329.

Lion T, Haas OA, Harbott J, et al. The translocation t(1;22) (p13;q13) is a nonrandom marker specifically associated with acute megakaryocytic leukemia in young children. Blood 1992;79:3325–3330.

Mazur E, Wittels EG, Schiffman FJ. Hand mirror cell lymphoid leukemia in adults: a distinct clinicopathologic syndrome. Case report and literature review. Cancer 1986;57:92–99.

Schumacher HR. Acute leukemia: approach to diagnosis. New York: Igaku-Shoin, 1990.

Schumacher HR, Cotelingam JD. Chronic leukemia: approach to diagnosis. New York: Igaku-Shoin, 1993.

Schumacher HR, Cotelingam JD, Hummer HK. Acute lymphoblastic leukemia. Cytochemistry and ultrastructure with emphasis on the hand mirror variant. In: Polliack A. Human leukemias. Boston: Martenus Nijhoff, 1984:219–250.

Sempere A, Jarque I, Guinot M, et al. Acute myeloblastic leukemia with minimal myeloid differentiation (FAB AML-M0): a study of eleven cases. Leuk Lymphoma 1993;12:103–108.

Sun T, Li CY, Yam LT. Atlas of cytochemistry and immunocytochemistry of hematologic neoplasm. Chicago: American Society of Clinical Pathology Press, 1985.

Tuzaner N, Cox C, Rowe JM, et al. Hypocellular acute myeloid leukemia: the Rochester (New York) experience. Hematol Pathol 1995;9:195–203.

van't Veer MB. The diagnosis of acute leukemia with undifferentiated or minimally differentiated blasts. Ann Hematol 1992;64:161–165.

Wibowo A, Pankowsky D, Mikhael A, et al. Adult acute leukemia: Hand mirror variant. Hematopathol Mol Hematol 1996;10:85–98.

Yamato H, Yamada K, Koike T, et al. Complete remission achieved by low-dose Ara-C, aclarubicin, and rhG-CSF (CAG) therapy in acute nonlymphocytic leukemia with monosomy 7 occurring after severe aplastic anemia. Rinsho Ketsueki 1995;36:128–133.

CHAPTER 3

Immunophenotype

GENERAL COMMENTS

Although the original emphasis for the diagnosis and classification of the acute leukemias was centered on morphology and cytochemistry, it became increasingly clear that the use of an appropriate panel of monoclonal antibodies for immunophenotyping was complementary in some cases and absolutely essential in others. By employing appropriate panels of monoclonal antibodies, it is possible to separate acute lymphoblastic leukemia (ALL) from acute myeloid leukemia (AML) with greater than 99% accuracy. The hallmark for lineage commitment is myeloperoxidase (MPEX) for myeloid lineage, and cytoplasmic CD22 and CD3 for B- and T-cell lineages, respectively. It is most important to note that CD22, CD3, and CD13 are expressed in the cytoplasm earlier than on the cell membrane, and that antibodies against MPEX have demonstrated greater sensitivity than conventional cytochemistry. Even though the FAB group has recognized the importance of immunophenotyping in FAB M0 and M7, they have not proposed using detailed immunologic data for separation of ALL and poorly differentiated AML. Contrariwise, other groups have utilized immunologic classifications of ALL in which discrete differentiation stages within either B- or T-cell lineage were identified by antigenic characteristics of the leukemic cells (Table 3.1).

B-lineage ALL has been classified by the Morphology, Immunology, Cytogenetics Cooperative Study Group (MIC) into four groups that are widely accepted. They include B precursor ALL (cCD22+, CD19+, TdT+, CD10−, cIg−, sIg−), common ALL (cCD22+, CD19+, TdT+, CD10+, cIg−, sIg−), pre B ALL (cCD22+, CD19+, TdT+, CD10+, cIg+, sIg−), and B ALL (cCD22+, CD19+, TdT−, CD10−, cIg−, sIg+). DeRossi et al. evaluated the immunophenotype of 304 adult lymphoblastic leukemias based on initial screening reactivity for TdT, HLA-DR, CD7, CD10, CD13, CD19, CD24, CD33, and CD41. According to results obtained, the second level of investigation assessed the positivity for intracytoplasmic (Cy) Ig, CD1a, CD2, CD3, CD4, CD5, CD8, and CD20. They classified the B-lineage ALL into five subgroups (B0 to B4) and the T-lineage ALL into four subgroups (T0 to T3).

The classification of T ALL is more controversial. Rheinhertz et al. proposed three stages: Stage I, early thymocytes express CD7, CD2, CD5, and CD71; Stage II, common thymocytes lose CD71 and acquire surface expression CD1, CD4, and CD8; and Stage III, medullary thymocytes lose CD1, express CD3, and retain either CD4 or CD8. Contrary to Rheinhertz and Foon, the MIC has suggested that T-cell ALL be divided into two categories: T precursor and T mature, on the basis of CD2 reactivity. This

Table 3.1
Immunophenotypic Leukemic Categories a,b

AML	HLA-DR	TdT	CD34	CD13	CD33	CD15	CD14	CD11b	CD41	Gly-A
M0	+	+/-	+	+/-	+/-	-/+	-/+	-/+	-	-
M1	+	+/-	+/-	+	+	-/+	-/+	-/+	-	-
M2	+	-/+	-/+	+	+	+	-/+	-/+	-	-
M3	-	-	-	+	+	+/-	-	-	-	-
M4	+	-/+	+/-	+	+	+	+	+	-	-
M5	+	-/+	+/-	+/-	+/-	+/-	+	+	-	-
M6	+/-	-	-/+	+/-	+/-	-	-/+	-/+	-	+
M7	+/-	-	+/-	-/+	-/+	-	-	-	+	-

B-lineage ALL	HLA-DR	TdT	CD34	CD19	CD24	CD10	CD20	CD22	clg	slg
Early B-precursor	+	+	+	+	+	-	-	-	-	-
Common	+	+	+/-	+	+	+	-/+	-	-	-
Pre-B	+	+	-/+	+	+	+	+	-	+	-
B-cell	+	-	-	+	+	+/-	+	+	+/-	+

T-lineage ALL	TdT	cCD3	CD7	cTCRβ	CD2	CD5	CD4	CD8	CD1	sCD3
Pro-thymocyte	+	+	+	–	–	–	–	–	–	–
Early T	+	+	+	+	+	+	–	–	–	–
Intermediate T	+	+	+	+	+	+	+	+	+	–
Mature T	–	(+)	+	(+)	+	+	+[c]	+[c]	–	+

From: Taylor CG, Stasi R, Bastianelli C, et al. Diagnosis and classification of the acute leukemias: recent advances and controversial issues. Hematopathol Molec Hematol 1996;10:1–38. Courtesy of Dr. Roberto Stasi.

[a] Only the most common patterns of reactivity are reported.

[b] +/– indicates that the marker is positive in the majority of cases; –/+ indicates that the marker is negative in the majority of cases. The parentheses indicate that only a subpopulation of these cells expresses this marker.

[c] CT mature T-lineage ALLs expressing CD4 do not express CD8, and vice versa.

Abbreviations: Gly-A, glycophorin-A; TdT, terminal deoxynucleotydil transferase; cIg, cytoplasmic immunoglobulin (μ chain); sIg, surface immunoglobulin; cCD3, cytoplasmic CD3; cTCRβ, cytoplasmic β chain of T cell receptor; sCD3, surface CD3.

classification has not been widely accepted. Others have divided the T ALLs into three groups based on membrane CD1 and CD3 reactivity. More T ALL cases need to be evaluated before a consensus can be solidified.

In contrast to T ALL, a consensus has been reached concerning immunologic analysis for AML. Immunophenotypic patterns tend to agree with morphology and cytochemistry. Few studies have identified phenotypes with exclusive distribution in a specific FAB or MIC category. In general, leukemic cells in AML almost universally express MPEX, surface CD13, and/or CD33 antigens (Table 3.1). Markers of hematopoietic precursor cells, such as TdT and CD34, tend to be expressed more frequently in blasts of FAB M0, M1, M5a. Also, HLA-DR is expressed on more immature cells, but continues to be found in subtypes with a higher degree of maturation with the exception of FAB M3, which is usually negative. CD4 and CD14 positivity is usually positive in cases with monocytic differentiation; whereas, CD15 antigen can be detected in the majority of cases of FAB M2, M4, and M5; in nearly half of M3 and M1 cases; and is almost always negative in M0. Recently, Macedo et al. investigated the immunophenotype of blast cells from 40 de novo AML patients at diagnosis with a large panel of monoclonal antibodies in double- and triple-staining combinations analyzed by flow cytometry. The differentiation associated antigens included CD34, CD117, HLA-DR, CD33, CD15, CD14, CD11b, and CD4. Interestingly, more than one blast cell subpopulation was identified in 34 patients (85%). Such lineage promiscuity or lineage infidelity has led to a plethora of terms including hybrid, biphenotypic, and mixed-lineage leukemia. These terms refer to a single blast that coexpresses different lineage associated markers; whereas, bilineage leukemia pertains to those cases where two distinct blast populations with different lineage features are identified. These unusual leukemias will be discussed in more detail later in this chapter.

ACUTE UNDIFFERENTIATED LEUKEMIA (AUL) (TABLE 3.2)

Since both morphology and cytochemistry (FAB criteria) are unable to classify this subtype of acute leukemia, some investigators have resorted to immunophenotypic analysis and molecular biology to diagnose or further subclassify this group. Campana et al. and Raimondi et al. have described 9 cases of 750 (1.2%) and 11 cases of 125 (8.8%) of acute leukemias as AUL, respectively. Interestingly, the former group defined AUL immunophenotypically as positive for any or all of the following antigens: CD34, HLA-DR, CD7, and TdT with absence of CD22, CD19, CD37, CD2, CD10, CD13, CD33, CD14, Glycophorin A, and CD61. The latter group's criteria, however, were less stringent using only nine monoclonal antibodies (CD2, CD5, CD7, CD10, CD19, CD20, CD13, CD33, and CD41) with the comment of reasonably low cost. No AUL in the Campana et al. series revealed T cell receptor (TCR) rearrangements, but two patients revealed rearrangements in Ig H.

Table 3.2
Summary of Immunophenotypes of Various Leukemias

Diagnosis FAB Subtype	Immunophenotype	Comment	References
AUL	Positive for any or all (CD34, HLA-DR, CD7, TdT). Negative for CD22, CD19, CD37, CD2, CD10, CD13, CD33, Glycophorin A, and CD61	Unclassified by all study parameters. RT-mRNA MPEX have classified some as myeloid	Leukemia 1990;4:620–624
Hypocellular/Aplastic ALL	No characteristic morphology, immuno-phynotype or cytogenetics. T-cell markers in some cases (CD2+, CD7+) TCR rearrangement	Complete remission with G-CSF in case reported from Japan	Acta Haematologica 1995;94:39–43 Pediat Hematol/Oncol 1995;17:270–275
Granular ALL	Early pre-B (CD10+, CIg−); Pre-B (CD10+, CIg+) T-cell (CD2+, CD3+, CD7+); coexpression of myeloid antigens (CD13+, CD33+)	B-cell precurson "common" immunophenotype predominates, but other lineages have been noted	Am J Clin Pathol 1991;95:526–531 Haematologica 1992;77:30–34
ALL with eosinophilia	B-lineage ALL. Immature T-cell lymphoma/myeloid leukemia reported. ATLL with eosinophilia CD2+, CD3+, CD4+, CD5+, CD8−, CD25+	Eosinophils not part of malignant clone. Stimulated by cytokines IL-3, IL-5, and GM-CSF	J Clin Oncol 1987;5:382–390 Am J Surg Path 1992;16:236–245
Acute leukemia with t(4;11)	Biphenotypic CD19+, CD24+/−, HLA-DR+, TdT+, CD10−, CD15+, CDw65+	Infants and young children—poor prognosis. ALL-1 locus on band 11q23 involved	Leuk Lymphoma 1992;7:173–179 Cancer Genet Cytogenet 1992;60:82–85
Acute leukemia-hand mirror variant (ALL-HMV)	Initially null, B, T, myeloid. Recently, biphenotypic with adhesion molecules present	Hand mirror morphology should alert clinician to biphenotypic leukemia with adhesion molecules. Such findings may help predict pathogenesis and initiate appropriate therapy	Am J Clin Path 1992;98:526–530 Hematopath Mol Hematol 1996;10:85–98
Aggressive natural killer cell leukemia (ANKCL)	CD3−, CD4−, CD16+, CD56+, CD71+, CD38+, CD2+, HLA-DR+	NK-LGL leukemias appear to be more aggressive than T-LGL leukemias. ANKCLs probably overlap with some of the NK-LGL leukemias in literature	Experimental Hematol 1996;24:406–415 Am J Hematol 1995;49:221–231

(Continued)

Table 3.2 *(Continued)*

Diagnosis FAB Subtype	Immunophenotype	Comment	References
AML-M0	Twenty percent or more blasts are positive for myeloid lineage-specific antibodies (CD13, CD14, CD33, MPEX). Lymphoid markers CD7 and TdT may be positive	Presence of CD34, multidrug resistance phenotype, complex karyotypes, gene rearrangements suggest origin from early hematopoietic precursor and reflected in a very poor prognosis	Hematopathol Mol Hematol 1996;10:1–38 Stem Cells 1995;13:428–434
AML-M6A, M6B Erythroleukemia	CD71, CD45, glycophorin positive in some cases. Glycophorin A mature marker and may miss immature cases. CD36 may be of value	Immunophenotypic analysis with markers capable of identifying immature erythroid elements may correctly place these cases into AML-M6B	Blood (letter) 1992;80:1097 Am J Hematol 1995;49:29–38
Acute basophilic leukemia (ABL)	No specific immunophenotype. Bsp-1 monoclonal antibody recognizes early basophils	Additional cases of basophilic leukemia need to be analyzed for immunophenotype by more specific antibodies	Cancer Genet Cytogenet 1989;42:209–219 Br J Haematol 1994;85:101–104
Eosinophilic leukemia (EL), hypereosinophilic syndrome (HES)	Limited data AML-M4Eo-inv(16) (p13q32) CD13+, partially positive CD2, CD11b, CD11c, CD14, CD33, CD34, CD36, CDw65, TdT, HLA-DR	Markers reflect myeloid population and not eosinophils per se. No good immunophenotypic studies available on leukemia eosinophils	Blood 1993;81: 3034–3051
Hypocellular AML	AML-M0-HLA-DR+ CD34, CD13+/–, CD33+/–, CD15–/+. TdT+/– AML-M1 HLA-DR+, CD13+, CD33+, AML HMZ HLA-DR+, CD134, CD33+, CD15+. Others variably +/–, –/+. See Table 3.1	Usually AML-M0, AML-M1, or AML-M2	Hematopathol Mol Hematol 1996;10:1–38
CD7 Positive AML	HLA-DR+, CD34+, TdT+,	Wide divergence of data. Needs additional evaluation	Lymphoma 1995;17:111–119 Pediat Hematol Oncol 1995;12:463–469 Blood 1986;68:406–411
AML 3(q21;q26)	AML-M1 HLA-DR+, CD13+, CD33+. AML-M4 HLA-DR+, CD13+, CD33+, CD15+, CD14+, CD11b. AML-M6-Glycophorin A+ (mature erythroid). Other markers variable. See Table 3.1	Variability in AML-M6 depending on number of myeloblasts and proerythroblasts. Glycophorin A not good marker for immature erythroid cells	Atlas tumor pathol: tumors bone marrow third series. Fascicle 1993;9:85

(Continued)

Table 3.2   *(Continued)*

Diagnosis FAB Subtype	Immunophenotype	Comment	References
Myeloid/NK leukemia	CD33+, CD56+, CD11a+, CD13 (dim), CD15 (dim), CD34+/−, HLA-DR-, CD16-	Important subtype to distinguish from AML-M3-M3v as it does not respond to ATRA	Blood 1994;84:244–255
Biphenotypic bilineage acute leukemia	Single leukemic cell expresses markers from different lineages (biphenotypic) or two different separate leukemic lineages exist (bilineage). See Tables 3.3, 3.4, and 3.5	No general acceptance of any criteria. Criteria has changed within same group.	Leuk Lymphoma 1994;13(Suppl 1): 11–14 Acta Haematol 1991;62:16–21 Hematol/Oncol Clin NA 1990;4:767–794

ACUTE LYMPHOBLASTIC LEUKEMIA (ALL) (TABLE 3.2)

Hypocellular/Aplastic Acute Leukemia

Aplastic/hypoplastic ALL is a rare disorder. Initially, leukemic blasts may be difficult to identify; however, the aplastic/hypocellular phase is typically followed by apparent bone marrow recovery and evolving leukemia in a matter of weeks or a few months. Although there are no distinctive morphologic, immunophenotypic, or cytogenetic characteristics associated with the leukemic phase, Hatta et al. reported a case that was negative for MPEX and positive for T cell markers (CD2 and CD7). Intriguingly, the 23-year-old male obtained a complete remission with granulocyte-colony-stimulating factor (G-CSF) alone. Also, Ishikawa et al. described a boy with hypocellular ALL (23.6% lymphoblasts) that responded to G-CSF. They found rearrangement of the TCR delta gene in the leukemic cell DNA by Southern blot hybridization.

Granular ALL (Table 3.2)

Azurophilic granules may be observed in the cytoplasm of leukemic cells of children and adults with a low overall incidence of 1.8 to 7.6%. Although granular ALL has been generally associated with the B cell common phenotype and FAB L2 morphology, coexpression of myeloid antigens and ultrastructural positivity for MPEX in other cases seem to indicate phenotypic deviation. Cerezo et al. analyzed 1252 fully studied ALLs in children. They found 56 cases (4.5%) that were characterized by the presence of more than 5% marrow blasts with at least three clearly defined azurophilic granules. The frequency of the granular features did not differ among early pre B (4.3%), pre B (3.6%), and T (5.8%) ALL. No cases were identified among the 12 patients with B-ALL. They observed that complete remission rates were significantly lower for those with granular lymphoblasts, regardless of risk group, immunophenotype, or FAB type. Also, they observed that their findings suggested a relationship between granules and L2 morphologic findings in childhood ALL and conveyed a worse prognosis. As discussed earlier, controversy exists concerning significance of granules in ALL.

ALL with Eosinophilia (Table 3.2)

Hogan et al. reported a case of ALL with eosinophilia and reviewed the literature at that time. Their patient, a 19-year-old man had ALL FABL2 with 82×10^9/L white blood cells, 57% eosinophils, and cardiorespiratory symptoms. Immunophenotyping, which was primitive by modern standards, revealed SmIg−, E-rosette−, OKT3−, OKT4−, and OKT8−.

Although the authors classified the case as a FAB L2 non B- non-T, the case most likely was of B-lineage.

T-cell lymphoblastic lymphoma and peripheral blood eosinophilia have been reported by Abruzzo et al. These cases demonstrated immature T-cell immunophenotype, and terminated with AML or granulocytic sarcoma. Similar cases have been reported with a t(8;13)(p11;q11) chromosomal abnormality. Although the authors referred to their two patients as having a distinctive biphenotypic hematologic disorder, the separate populations suggest a bilinear malignancy.

Adult T-cell leukemia/lymphoma (ATLL) may be associated with eosinophilia. These cases are mature T cells and are CD2+, CD3+, CD4+, CD5+, CD8−, and CD25+.

Acute Leukemia with t(4;11) (Table 3.2)

Patients with acute leukemia with t(4;11) have a unique immunophenotype in virtually all cases. The blast cells are CD19+, CD24+/−, HLA-DR+, TdT+ and CD10−. Many, but not all cases, express CD15+ and this phenotype is specific, as well as sensitive, for predicting 11q23 abnormalities. Besides CD15, CDw65 may also be expressed. Since many of these cases have overlapping lymphoid/myeloid surface markers, many investigators have referred to them as mixed-lineage leukemias, bilineage-biphenotypic, etc.

ALL-Hand Mirror Variant (HMV) (Table 3.2)

The initial reports on HMVs in leukemia described these cells in both acute lymphoblastic and myeloblastic leukemia. Shortly thereafter, a subset was described that was characterized by female predominance, null phenotype, acid phosphatase and TdT positivity, indolent course, and poor response to therapy. Unfortunately these cases were not investigated by current technology that would have allowed more detailed immunophenotypic and genotypic analysis of the hand mirror cells (HMCs) in those cases.

More recent studies of other cases of acute leukemia revealed biphenotypic features different from the initial ALL-HMV subset. Kovarik et al. reported on a female patient that initially appeared to be an ALL-HMV, but on further study demonstrated a mixed lineage. Immunophenotyping of the bone marrow mononuclear cells in this case revealed high activity for HLA-DR (96%), CD33 (91%), CD11b (87%), CD15 (89%), CD34 (94%), and CD71 (71%). Significant reactivity was also observed for CD13 (49%), CD11c (25%), PLT1 (42%), CD19 (70%), and CD25 (24%). Two color analysis showed simultaneous expression of TdT and CD19, TdT and CD33, and CD19 and CD33. Cytogenetic studies revealed a t(11;19) previously described in biphenotypic leukemias. Also, cases of acute mixed lineage leukemia in children show a high number of HMCs. Zucker et al. described an acute biphenotypic leukemia with mixed blast morphology and HMCs. The blast cells showed combined myeloid and T-lymphoid features. They noted that their case was similar to cases of biphenotypic leukemia described previously in children. Recently, Wibowo et al. described two patients with HMCs and mixed immunophenotype with expression of myeloid and T-lymphoid features. Interestingly, the blast cells showed strong expression of adhesive molecules CD2 and CD11b. Review of the above mixed leukemias with HMCs revealed they all expressed adhesion molecules. Most recently, we have observed a mixed leukemia with HMCs expressing CD56 (N-CAM) and central nervous system involvement. Such cases emphasize the importance of carefully evaluating cases with HMV morphology.

Aggressive NK Cell Leukemia (ANKCL) (Table 3.2)

Large granular lymphocytosis (LGL) leukemia can be divided into two large groups; T-LGL and NK-LGL. The former group is CD3+ whereas the latter group is CD3−. T-LGL are usually CD3+, CD4−, CD8+, CD16+, CD56−, CD57+, and often HLA-DR+. NK-LGL leukemias are usually CD3−, CD4−, CD8−, CD16+, CD56+, and CD57−. Undoubtedly there is some overlap between NK-LGL leukemia and ANKCL; however, the patients with ANKCL have abnormal cells that express an activated T-cell marker (CD38) and a marker for proliferating cells (CD71).

Recently, Robertson et al. established a cell line from a patient with ANKCL. The leukemic cells were obtained from the peripheral blood and were CD3−, CD16+, and CD56+. They mediated natural killing and antibody-dependent cellular cytotoxicity and exhibited proliferative responses similar to normal CD16+ CD56 dim NK cells. The NK leukemia cells expressed CD2, CD6, CD11a, CD26, CD27, CD29, CD38, CD43, CD58, CD81, CD94, CD95, and class II MHC. They did not express CD3, CD4, CD5, CD8, CD14, CD19, CD20, CD28, alpha/beta or gamma/delta TCRs on the cell surface. Such cell lines may prove useful for studies of human NK cell biology and give insights into therapeutic approaches.

ACUTE MYELOID LEUKEMIA (AML) (TABLE 3.2)

AML M0

The diagnosis of this FAB subtype is heavily dependent on immunopheno-typing and/or transmission electron microscopy. Less than 3% of the blasts are positive for MPEX and SBB and, in most cases, no or only rare blasts are positive; however, 20% or more blasts are reactive with one or more myeloid lineage specific antibody MPEX, CD13, CD14, CD33. Lymphoid markers are negative with the exception of CD7 and TdT. The TdT positivity is usually less than that observed in most cases of ALL. Since the cells of the AML M0 are very primitive, most of the cases express CD34 and HLA-DR. Also, the multidrug resistance gene can be found in the majority of the cases.

Recently, Lauria et al. evaluated 110 adult patients with a diagnosis of AML using a wide panel of monoclonal antibodies. Fifty-one percent expressed only myeloid antigens; whereas, 49% expressed both myeloid and lymphoid antigens. CD13 and CD33 were expressed in almost all FAB AML subtypes, whereas CD14, frequently expressed in AML M4 and M5 subtypes, was rarely expressed in AML M0 and M1 cases (9%). Contrariwise, CD34 expressed in 77% of AML M0 and M1 cases was practically absent in AML M3 and M5 subtypes. CD2 and CD7 antigens were found in 34% and 42% of AML patients, respectively. B-cell-associated antigens such as CD10 and CD19 were found in 31% and 18% of the patients, respectively. The only prognostic significance noted was represented by CD34+ patients who showed a reduction in the complete remission rate compared with CD34− patients. This became even more evident when the mean intensity of fluorescence was considered.

AML M6-Erythroleukemia (Table 3.2)

Immunophenotyping of the erythroleukemias has been used by Loken et al. They used glycophorin, the transferrin receptor (CD71), and the leukocyte common antigen (CD45); however, Maynadie et al. noted that the glycophorin A may be negative in some AML M6 cases since it represents a relatively mature marker. In analysis of two cases they observed an increased CD71 with decreased expression of CD34 and HLA-DR. Glycophorin A was only expressed in 27% and 20% of the erythroid cells. Furthermore, they suggest that acute leukemia secondary to MDS should lead to a more systematic search for CD34 and CD71 expression. Such analysis may undercover the underestimation of M6 acute MDS transformation and allow for the diagnosis of more AML M6B. San Miguel et al. have not only used glycophorin A and CD71, but also CD36 to uncover the broadest spectrum possible within erythroid differentiation in view of the absence of specific early erythroid markers. Davey et al. studied the clinical, morphologic, immunophenotypic, and cytogenetic features of 52 patients with erythroleukemia. They found that 50% or more of cases studied were positive for CD11b, CD13, CD15, CD33, glycophorin-A, and HLA-DR markers. They concluded that AML M6 is typified by multilineage involvement of hematopoietic cells.

Acute Basophilic Leukemia (ABL) (Table 3.2)

Diagnosis of basophilic leukemia is usually not decided by immunophenotypic analysis. ABL must be distinguished from AML M1, AML M0, and ALL. Such distinction may not be possible by routine cytochemical stains and immunologic markers. Any evidence of basophilic maturation in a poorly differentiated leukemia that is MPEX, SBB and nonspecific esterase, and TdT negative should suggest ABL. The definitive evidence is at the ultrastructural level in difficult cases.

Recently, Harada et al. reported on three cases of acute leukemia with t(4;12)(q11-12;p13). All three showed dysplasia of three hematopoietic lineages, absent or low peroxidase, and retention of platelets in the peripheral blood and megakaryocytes in the bone marrow. Increased numbers of basophils were observed in the blood and bone marrow of two cases. The blast cells displayed a unique immunophenotype CD7+, CD13+, CD34+, HLA-DR+. One case expressed c-kit (CD117) on the membrane surface. Although ultrastructural studies were not performed, the pronounced basophilia in both peripheral blood and bone marrow suggested a basophilic leukemia. Erber et al. reported 21 cases of AML M3 with characteristic myeloid phenotype, coexpression of CD9 and CD68 antigens and absence of HLA-DR. They stated that the phenotype of acute promyelocytic leukemia is similar to that of basophils and mast cells and raised the possibility that the leukemic cells may have undergone a degree of basophilic differentiation. Although the above immunophenotypic analyses were performed in cases associated with basophils, none of the markers are specific for basophilic lineage. Nevertheless, Cuneo et al. have used immunolabeling with monoclonal antibody Bsp-1 and electron microscopy to recognize early basophilic differentiation.

Eosinophilic Leukemia (EL)/Hypereosinophilic Syndrome (HES) (Table 3.2)

Few immunophenotypic studies have been performed on malignant eosinophils or on diseases that are associated with malignant eosinophils. However, Adriaansen et al. performed extensive immunophenotypic analysis on eight patients with AML M4Eo with inv(16) (p13q32). The eight cases consisted of heterogeneous cell populations; mainly due to the presence of multiple subpopulations, which varied in size between the patients. Nevertheless, the immunophenotype of these subpopulations was comparable, independent of their relative sizes. Virtually all AML M4Eo cells were positive for the pan-myeloid marker CD13. In addition, the leukemic cells were partly positive for CD2, CD11b, CD11c, CD14, CD33, CD34, CD36, CDw65, TdT, and HLA-DR. Double immunofluorescence stainings demonstrated coexpression of the CD2 antigen and myeloid markers and allowed the recognition of multiple AML subpopulations. The CD2 antigen was expressed by immature AML cells (CD34+, CD14−) and more mature monocytic AML cells (CD34−, CD14+); whereas, TdT expression was exclusively found in the CD34+, CD14−, cell population. The eight AML M4Eo cases not only expressed the CD2 antigen, but also its ligand CD58 (leukocyte function antigen-3). The high expression of CD2 in AML M4Eo stimulates proliferation of the leukemic cells, which might explain the high white blood cell count often found in this type of AML.

Significant immunophenotypic studies on the eosinophils from eosinophilic leukemia and the hyper-eosinophilic syndrome are not recoverable from the literature by Medline search; however, eosinophils are known to release superoxide, H_2O_2, and to express receptors for IgG, and IgE, IgA, C1q, C3b/4b(CR1), iC3b (CR3), C5a, IL3, IL5, granulocyte-macrophage colony-stimulating factor (GM-CSF), platelet activating factor, leukotriene B4, estrogens, and glycocorticoids. Additionally, eosinophils express the leukocyte adhesion glycoproteins LFA-1 (CD11a), CR3(CD11b) and gp 150/95 (CD11c); and the common beta chain CD18. Mature eosinophils retain the ability to synthesize CD4 and HLA-DR, and may form new proteins relevant to immunologic demands. However, the precise mechanism involved in the interaction of eosinophils with neoantigens remains to be elucidated.

Hypocellular AML (Table 3.2)

This subtype of AML does not define a specific cytologic type, but the majority of cases are AML M0, AML M1 or AML M2. The AML M0s are HLA-DR+, CD34+, CD13+/-, CD33+/-, CD15-/+, CD14-/+, CD11b-/+ and TdT+/-. It also may react with the myeloid-specific antibody MPEX and may be positive for ultrastructural MPEX. The AML M1s are HLA-DR+, CD34+/-, CD13+, CD33+, CD15-/+, CD14-/+, CD11b-/+ and TdT+/-. The AML M2s are HLA-DR+, CD13+, CD33+, CD15+, CD34-/+, CD15-/+, CD14-/+, CD11-/+ and TdT-/+. Blasts in 40% to 80% of t(8;21) associated AML M2 cases are CD19 positive. Also, approximately 20% of these cases are TdT+.

CD7 Positive AML (Table 3.2)

Some investigators have found adverse prognostic significance to CD7+ AML; however, recently, Kornblau et al. analyzed CD7 expression by flow cytometric analysis using the Leu 9 monoclonal antibody in 331 patients with newly diagnosed AML. There was a marked imbalance in the distribution of favorable cytogenetic abnormalities t(8;21), inv 16, t(15;17), with 95% segregating to the CD7-group. Analysis excluding patients with favorable cytogenetic abnormalities revealed no prognostic importance for CD7 expression. They further showed that the response rate, survival experiences of CD7+ and CD7− patients were similar with six different treatment regimens. In further support of these findings, Kawai et al. in analysis of 66 children with newly diagnosed AML found 17% were CD7+, 15% were CD19+, 8% were CD2+, and 5% were CD10+. Chromosomal analysis revealed t(8;21) in 6 of the 21 Ly+AML cases examined. No other specific chromosome aberration was noted. Most recently, Del Poeta et al. have suggested that CD7 expression is associated with abnormal complex karyotypes. They found no significant difference between the 23 Ly+ and 43 Ly− AML cases. From the wide divergence of data in CD7+AML, it would appear that conflicting results most likely relate to the methodology used by various investigators and evaluation of cytogenetics in light of immunophenotypic data. Additional future well-designed studies are needed to more clearly resolve this issue.

AML 3(q21;q26) (Table 3.2)

AMLs associated with these abnormalities are difficult to classify by morphology. Reported cases have included AML M1, AML M4, and AML M6. The AML M1s are HLA-DR+, CD13+, CD33+, CD34+/−, CD15-/+, CD14−/+, CD11b−/+, and TdT+/-. The AML M4s are HLA-DR+, CD13+, CD33+, CD15+, CD14+, CD11b+, CD C34-/+, and TdT−/+. The AML M6 are glycophorin A+/−, HLA-DR+, CD13+/−, CD33+/−, CD34−/+, CD14−/+, CD11b−/+, CD15−, and TdT−. The immunophenotype of the AML M6 will vary depending on the numbers of myeloblasts and/or proerythroblasts present. Also, as mentioned previously, the detection of glycophorin A on the surface of immature erythroid series is not a satisfactory technique for identifying those cases with immature erythroid elements.

The AML cases with 3(q21;q26) have been associated with a poor prognosis. They generally are associated with abnormalities of megakaryocytopoiesis, including micromegakaryocytes and increased megakaryocytes.

Myeloid/NK-Leukemia (Table 3.2)

These cases represent an important subset that has been confused with AML M3, especially the microgranular variant. Scott et al. identified 20 (6%) of 350 cases of adult de novo AML with this unique subtype. In the past, these cases were most likely misdiagnosed as AML M3 or AML M3v. They express the exclusive immunophenotype: CD33+, CD56+, CD1/a+, CD13 (dim), CD15(dim), CD34+/−, HLA-DR−, CD16−. Multicolor flow cytometric analysis confirmed the coexpression of myeloid (CD33, CD13,

CD15) and NK cell associated (CD56) antigens in all the cases studied. Although two cases expressed CD4, none showed CD2, CD3, or CD8 expression on their cells. Four of six cases tested revealed functional NK cell-mediated cytotoxicity, suggesting a relationship between these unique CD33+, CD56+, CD16− acute leukemias and normal CD56+, CD16−, NK precursor cells.

Of interest and importance is that none of these six cases were capable of differentiation in vitro in response to all-transretinoic acid (ATRA). Such findings may account for the fact that some AML M3s (misdiagnosed) have not shown a clinical response to ATRA.

BILINEAGE/BIPHENOTYPIC ACUTE LEUKEMIA (TABLE 3.2)

As noted in Chapter 1, one of the greatest problems in dealing with this group of leukemias is terminology. As stated previously, the term biphenotypic leukemia should be confined to those cases when coexpression of lymphoid and myeloid markers occurs on the same cells. On the other hand, bilineage leukemia demonstrates the presence of two blast populations: one showing myeloid morphology and immunophenotype, and the other displaying lymphoid morphology and immunophenotype.

Difficulties arise because many immunologic markers utilized in routine immunophenotyping are usually lineage associated rather than lineage specific. This resulted because detailed analysis of normal cell lineages and tissues revealed a much broader extent of antigenic distribution as compared to initial observations. Examples include TdT and CD7 which appear early during hematopoietic ontogeny and are found on precursors of both lymphoid and myeloid cells. Therefore, it is not surprising that their expression in leukemic cells is less restricted than crucial cytoplasmic markers such as MPEX, CD3, CD22. The occurrence of ectopic antigen expression in acute leukemia is extremely variable, depending on the panel of monoclonal antibodies utilized, techniques, and equipment. The presence of lymphoid-associated antigens in AML shows wide variability from 2% to 60% of cases. Contrariwise, myeloid antigen expression in ALL appears to vary with age, approaching 35% in adults, and ranging from 3.5% to 20% in children.

In an attempt to establish a comprehensive scheme for diagnosis, Hurwitz and Mirro used morphologic, cytochemical, immunologic, and karyotypic data (Tables 3.3 and 3.4). Note that the expression of a single inappropriate antigen did not permit the establishment of a lineage, but a minimum of two or more points from each category are required to classify the case as biphenotypic. Catovsky et al. proposed a scoring system based mostly on immunophenotypic findings and IgH and TCR rearrangement analysis (Table 3.5). Initially, the minimum score of 2 from two separate lineages has been increased to 2.5. Of 180 patients most "true" biphenotypic cases scored between 2.5 and 5. Finally, this group further modified their criteria by excluding data of rearrangement of lymphocyte functional genes, because of

Table 3.3
Criteria for the Diagnosis of Biphenotypic Leukemia[a]

Lymphoid Criteria	Points
Cytoplasmic Ig[b]	2.0
Surface Ig	2.0
Ig light chain gene rearrangement	2.0
Karyotypic abnormalities (see Table 3)	2.0
37°C E-rosette formation	2.0
Surface TCR[c] expression (WT-31)	2.0
Ig heavy chain gene rearrangement	1.0
TdT[d] expression	1.0
TCR gene rearrangements (gamma or beta)	1.0
CD19, CD20, CD21	1.0
CD22 (cytoplasmic or surface) expression	1.0
CD3 (cytoplasmic or surface) expression	1.0
CD5 or CD8 expression	1.0

Myeloid Criteria	
Myeloperoxidase (>3% by light or electron microscopy)	2.0
Auer rods	2.0
Alpha naphthyl butyrate	2.0
Platelet peroxidase	2.0
Karyotypic abnormalities (see Table 1.3)	2.0
10F7, CD41 or CD42d expression	2.0
Sudan black B	1.0
CD13 or CD33 or CD14, or CD15, or Leu 19 expression	1.0

From Hematol/Oncol/Clin NA 1990;4:767–794.

[a] Two or more points from each category are needed.
[b] Immunoglobulin.
[c] T-cell receptor.
[d] Terminal deoxynucleotidyl transferase.

the high incidence of IgH and TCR gene rearrangement observed in AML with expression of lymphoid markers. In this scheme they utilize a monoclonal antibody specific for the Ig-linked mb-1 polypeptide (Table 3.6). Their results reveal that mb-1 is a sensitive and specific reagent for B-lineage blasts that will aid in the classification of B-cell precursor ALL and in the identification of biphenotypic leukemia presenting as AML. In this scheme, a score of greater than 2 points for the myeloid and one lymphoid lineage are required.

The latest information on cluster designation (CD) antigens is depicted in Table 3.7.

Table 3.4
Karyotypic Abnormalities That are Strongly Lineage Associated

Cytogenetic Abnormality	Associated Immunologic or Morphologic Type of Leukemia
t(7;12)(q11;p12)	B lineage
dic(9;12)(p11;p12)	B lineage
t(12;V)(p12;V)[a]	B lineage
t(9;22)(q34;q11)	B lineage
t(1;19)(q23;p13.3)	Pre B
t(8;14)(Q24;Q32)	B Cell
t(8;22)(q24;q11)	B Cell
t(2;8)(p12;q24)	B Cell
t(11;14)(p13;q11)	T lineage
t(8;14)(q24;q11)	T lineage
t(10;14)(q24;q11)	T lineage
t(1;14)(p32;q11)	T lineage
t(7;V)(q32-q36;V)	T lineage
inv(14)(q11q32)	T lineage
t(8;21)(q22;q22)	FAB-M2
t(15;17)(q22;q12)	FAB-M3 or M3v
inv(16)(p13q22)/del(16)(q22)	FAB-M4 Eo, or M2
t(9;22)(q34;q11)	FAB-M1 or M2
t(6;9)(p23;q34)	FAB-M2 or M4 with basophilia
t(9;11)(p21-p22;q23)	FAB-M5 or M4
t(11;V)(q23;V)	FAB-M5 or M4
t(3;5)(q25.1;q34)	Preleukemia, M2, M6
t(8;16)(p11p13)	FAB-M5b
inv(3)(q21q26)	FAB-M1 (M2, M4, M7) with thrombocytosis
−7/7q−	FAB-M1 through M5
5q−	FAB-M1 through M4

From Hematol/Oncol Clin NA 1990;4:767–794.

[a] V indicates a variable chromosome.

Table 3.5
Scoring System for Biphenotypic Acute Leukemia[a]

Points	B-lineage	T-lineage	Myeloid Lineage
2	cCD22	cCD3	MPO (any method including Anti-MPO)[b]
	cμ chain		
1	CD10	CD2	CD33
	CD19	CD5	CD13 m/c
	CD24	TCR rearr	CD14 m/c
		(β or δ chain)	AML morphology or cytochemistry
			(other than MPO)[c]
0.5	TdT	TdT	CD11b
	IgH rearr	CD7	CD11c
			CD15

From Ann Hematol 1991;62:16–21.

[a] Two or more points from 2 separate lineages are required to classify a case as biphenotypic AL. Most biphenotypic AL have a mixture of myeloid and lymphoid (B or T) markers; exceptionally, cases with coexpression B and T markers have been reported.

[b] Cases suspected of being myeloid, but with negative MPO by light microscopy cytochemistry or anti-MPO by MoAb need analysis by electron microscopy.

[c] Diffuse/strong alpha naphthyl esterase (ANAE) sensitive to sodium fluoride and/or positive Sudan black B.

Table 3.6
Scoring System for the Definition of Acute Biphenotypic Leukemia[a]

Score Points	B-lymphoid	T-lymphoid	Myeloid
2	mb-1	CD3	MPO
	cyt CD22		
	cyt IgM		
1.5	CD19	CD2	CD13
	CD10	CD5	CD33
1	TdT	TdT	CD14
		CD7	CD11b
			CD11c

From Leuk Lymphoma 1994;13(suppl 1):11–14.

[a] A case is defined biphenotypic when scores > 2 points for the myeloid and one lymphoid lineage.

Table 3.7a
CD Antigens[a]

CD Design	Selection of Assigned Monoclonal Antibodies	Main Cellular Reactivity	Recognized Membrane Component[b]	Sequenced CH-Structure Analyzed[c]
CD1a	NA 1/34; T6 VIT6; Leu6	Thy, DC, B subset	gp49	Y
CD1b	WM-25; 4A76; NUT2	Thy, DC, B subset	gp45	Y
CD1c	L161; M241; 7C6; PHM3	Thy, DC, B subset	gp43	Y
CD2	9.6; T11; 35.1	T	CD58 (LFA-3) receptor, gp50	Y
CD2R	T11.3; VIT 13; D66	Activated T	CD2 epitopes restr. to activ. T	Y
CD3	T3; UCHT1; 38.1; Leu4	T	CD3-complex (5 chains), gp/p 26,20,16	Y
CD4	T4; Leu3a;91.D6	T subset	Class II/HIV receptor, gp59	Y
CD5	T1; UCHT2; T101; HH9; AMG4	T, B subset	gp67	Y
CD6	T12; T411	T, B subset	gp100	—
CD7	3A1; 4A; CL1.3; G3-7	T	gp40	Y
CD8	α chain: T8; Leu2a; M236; UCHT4; T811 β chain: T8/2T8-5H7	T subset	Class I receptor, gp 32α, /or/ β dimer	Y
CD9	CLB-thromb/8; PHN200; FMC56	Pre-B, M, Pit	p24	—
CD10	J5, VILA1, BA-3	Lymph. Prog., cALL, Germ. Ctr. B, G	Neutral endopeptidase, gp100, CALLA	Y
CD11a	MHM24; 2FI2; CRIS-3	Leukocytes	LFA-1, gp180/95	Y
CD11b	Mo1; 5A4.C5; LPM19C	M, G, NK	C3bi receptor, gp155/95	—
CD11c	B-LY6; L29; BL-4H4	M, G, NK, B sub	gp150/95	—
CDw12	M67	M, G, Pit	(p90-120)	—
CD13	MY7, MCS-2, TÜK1, M0U28	M, G	Aminopeptidase N, pg150	Y
CD14	Mo2, UCHM1, VIM13, MoP15	M, (G), LHC	gp55	Y
CD15	My1, VIM-D5	G, (M)	3-FAL, X-Hapten	Y
CD16	BW209/2; HUNK2; VEP13; 3G8	NK, G, Mac	FcRIII, gp50-65	Y
CDw17	GO35, Huly-m 13	G, M, Pit	Lactosylcaramide	—
CD18	MHM23; M232; 11H6; GLB54	Leukocytes	β chain to CD11a,b,c	Y
CD19	B4; HD37	B	gp95	Y
CD20	B1; 1F5	B	p37/32, ion channel?	Y
CD21	B2, HB5	B subset	C3d/EBV-Rec. (CR2), p140	Y
CD22	HD39; S-HCL1; To15	Cytopl. B/surface B subset	gp135, homology to myelin assoc. gp (MAG)	Y

Table 3.7a *(Continued)*

CD Design	Selection of Assigned Monoclonal Antibodies	Main Cellular Reactivity	Recognized Membrane Component[b]	Sequenced CH-Structure Analyzed[c]
CD23	Blast-2, MHM6	B subset, act M, Eo	FceRII, gp45-50	Y
CD24	VIBE3; BA-1	B, G	gp41/38?	—
CD25	TAC; 7G7/B6;2A3	Activated T, B, M	IL-2R βchain, gp55	Y
CD26	134-2C2; TS145	Activated T	Dipeptidylpeptidase IV, gp 120	Y
CD27	VIT14; S152; OKT18A; CLB-9F	T subset	p55 (dimer)	—
CD28	9.3; KOLT2	T subset	gp44	Y
CD29	K20; A-1A5	Broad	VLA β-, integrin β1-chain, Plt GPIIa	Y
CD30	Ki-1; Ber-H2; HSR4	Activated T, B; Sternberg-Reed	gp120, Ki-1	—
CD31	SG134; TM3; HEC-75; ES12F11	Pit, M, G, B, (T)	gp140, Plt GPIIa	—
CDw32	CIKM5; 41H16; IV.3; 2E1; KB61	M, G, B, Plt	FcRII, gp40	Y
CD33	My9; H153; L4F3	M, Prog., AML	gp67	Y
CD34	MY10, BI-3C5, ICH-3	Prog.	gp105-120	Y
CD35	TO5, CB04, J3D3	G, M, B	CR1	Y
CD36	5F1, C1MEG1; ESIVC7	M, Plt, (B)	gp90, Plt GPIV	—
CD37	HD28; HH1; G28-1	B, (T, M)	gp40-52	Y
CD38	HB7; T16	Lymph, Prog., PC Act. T	p45	Y
CD39	AC2; G28-2	B subset, (M)	gp70-100	—
CD40	G28-5	B, carcinomas	gp50, homology to NGF-receptor	Y
CD41	PBM 6.4; CLB-thromb/7; PL273	Plt	Plt GPIIb/IIIa complex and GPIIb	Y
CD42a	FMC25; BL-H6; GR-P	Plt	Plt GPIX, gp23	Y
CD42b	PHN89; AN51; GN287	Plt	Plt GPIb, gp135/25	Y
CD43	OTH 71C5; G19-1; MEM-59	T, G, M, brain	Leukosialin, gp95	Y
CD44	GRHL 1; F10-44-2; 33-3B4; BRIC35	T, G, M, brain, RBC	Pgp-1, gp80-95	Y
CD45	T29/33; BMAC 1; AB187	Leukocytes	LCA, T200	Y
CD45RA	G1-15; F8-11-13; 73.5	T subset, B, G, M	Restricted T200, gp220	Y
CD45RB	PTD/26/16	T subset, B, G, M	Restricted T200,	Y
CD45RO	UCHL 1	T subset, B, G, M	Restricted T200, gp180	Y
CD46	HULYM5; 122-2; J4B	Leukocytes	MCP, gp66/56	Y
CD47	BRIC 126; CIKM1; BRIC 125	Broad	gp47-52, *N*-linked glycan	—
CD48	WM68; LO-MN25; J4-57	Leukocytes	gp41, PI-linked	—

Table 3.7a (*Continued*)

CD Design	Selection of Assigned Monoclonal Antibodies	Main Cellular Reactivity	Recognized Membrane Component[b]	Sequenced CH-Structure Analyzed[c]
CD49b	CLB-thromb/4; Gi14	Plt, cultured T	VLA-alpha2-chain, Plt GPIa	Y
CDw49d	B5G10; HP2/1; HP1/3	M, T, B, (LHC), Thy	VLA-alpha4-chain, gp150	—
CDw49f	GoH3	Plt, (T)	VLA-alpha6-chain, Plt GPIc	—
CDw50	101-1D2; 140-11	Leukocytes	gp148/108, PI-linked	—
CD51	13C2; 23C6; NKI-M7; NKI-M9	(Plt)(B)	VNR α chain	Y
CDw52	097; YTH66.9; Campath-1	Leukocytes	Campath-1, gp21-28	
CD53	MEM-53; HI29 HI36; HD77	Leukocytes	gp32-40	—
CD54	RR7/7F7; WEHI-CAMI	Broad, Activ.	ICAM-1	Y
CD55	143-30; BRIC 110:BRIC 128; F2B-7.2	Broad	DAF (decay accelerating factor), PI-linked	Y
CD56	Leu19; NKH1; FP2-11.14, L185	NK, activ. lympho-cytes	gp220/135, NKH1, isoform of N-CAM	Y
CD57	Leu7; L183; L186	NK, T, B sub, brain	gp110, HNK1	—
CD58	TS2/9; G26; BRIC 5	Leukocytes, Epithel	LFA-3, gp40-65, PI-linked	Y
CD59	YTH53.1; MEM-43	Broad	gp18-20, PI-linked	—
CDw60	M-T32; M-T21; M-T41; UM4D4	T sub	NeuAc-Neu Ac-Gal	Y
CD61	Y2/51; CLB-thromb/1; VI-PL2; BL-E6	Plt	Integrin β3-,VNR β-chain, Plt GPIIIa	Y
CD62	CLB-thromb/6; CLB-thromb/5; RUU-SP1.18.1	Plt activ.	CMP-140 (PADGEM), gp140	Y
CD63	RUU-SP2.28; CLB-gran/12	Plt activ., M, (G, T, B)	gp53	—
CD64	Mab32.2; Mab22	M	FcRI, gp75	Y
CDw65	VIM2; HE10; CF4 VIM8	G, M	Ceramide-dodecasaccharide 4c	
CD66	CLB gran/10; YTH71.3	G	Phosphoprotein pp 180-200	—
CD67	B13.9; G10F5; JML-H16	G	p100, PI-linked	—
CD68	EBM11; Y2/131; Y-1/82A; Ki-M7; Ki-M6	Macrophages	gp110	—
CD69	MLR3; L78; BL-Ac/p26; FN50	Activated B, T	gp32/28, AIM	—
CDw70	Ki-24; HNE 51; HNC 142	Activated B, T, Sternberg-Reed cells	Ki-24	—
CD71	138-18; 120-2A3; MEM-75; VIP-1; Nu-TfR2	Proliferating cells, Mac.	Transferrin receptor	Y
CD72	S-HCL2; J3-109; BU-40; BU-41	B	gp43/39	—

Table 3.7a *(Continued)*

CD Design	Selection of Assigned Monoclonal Antibodies	Main Cellular Reactivity	Recognized Membrane Component[b]	Sequenced CH-Structure Analyzed[c]
CD73	1E9.28.1; 7G2.2.11 AD2	B subset, T subset	ecto-5'-nucleotidase p69	—
CD74	LN2; BU-43; BU-45	B, M	Class II assoc. invariant chain, gp41/35/33	—
CDw75	LN1; HH2; EBU-141	Mature B, (T subset)	p53?	—
CD76	HD66; CRIS-4	Mature B, T subset	gp85/67	—
CD77	38.13(BLA); 424/ 4A11; 424/3D9	Restr. B	Globotriaosylceramide (Gb3)	—
CDw78	Anti Ba; LO-panB-a; 1588	B, (M)	?	

Source: Knapp W et al, eds. Leukocyte typing IV. White cell differentiation antigens. New York: Oxford University Press, 1989. From Schlossman SF, Boumsell L, Gilks W, et al. CD antigens 1993 (commentary). Blood 1994; 83:879–880.

[a] Members of the Nomenclature Committee of the Fourth International Workshop on Human Leukocyte Differentiation Antigens: *Workshop Council:* A. Bernard, P. Beverley, L. Bournsell, T. Kishimoto, W. Knapp, A. McMichael, C. Milstein, S.F. Schlossman, E. Reinherz, G. Riethmüller, T.A. Springer, R. Winchester. *Workshop Organizers: T-Cell Section:* P. Rieber, R. Kurrle, S. Meuer. *B-Cell Section:* B. Dörken, G. Moldenhauer, P. Möller, A. Pezzutto, R. Schwartz-Albiez. *Myeloid Antigen Section:* W. Knapp, P. Bettelheim, S. Gadd, U. Köller, O. Majdic, C. Peschel, T. Radaszkiewicz, H. Stockinger, P.A.T. Tetteroo, C. E.v. d. Schoot. *Nk-/NL-Section:* R.E. Schmidt, A.C. Feller, M.R. Hadam, J. Johnson, J. Schubert, R. Schwinzer, M. Stoll, P. Uciechowski, K. Wonigeit. *Activation Antigen Section:* H. Stein, R. Schwarting. *Platelet Section:* A.E.G.Kr.v.d. Borne, L.G. de Bruijne-Admiraal, P.W. Modderman, H.K. Nieuwenhuis. *Statistics Section:* W.R. Gilks, L. Oldfield, A. Rutherford.

[b] Abbreviations: Thy, thymocytes; DC, dendritic cells; B, B cells; T, T cells; M, monocytes; MCP, membrane cofactor protein; G, granulocytes; Plt, platelets; Prog., progenitor cells; Germ. Ctr. B, germinal center B cells; NK, NK cells; Mac, macrophages; cytopl., cytoplasmic; LHC, epidermal Langerhans cells.

[c] Y, for protein antigens: sequence data available; for carbohydrate antigens: reactive oligosaccharide structure known.

Table 3.7b
CD Antigens[a]

CD Designation	Common Name	Workshop Section	MW Reduced	CD Designation	Common Name	Workshop Section	MW Reduced
CD15s	sLe, Sialyl Lewis	Adhesion		CD85	VMP-55, GH1/75	B cell	120,83
CD16	FcR IIIA/FcR IIIB	Myeloid	50-65	CD86	FUN-1, BU63	B cell	80
CD16b	FcR IIIB	Myeloid	48	CD87	UPA-R	Myeloid	50-65
CD32	Previously CDw32, FcRII	Myeloid	40	CD88	C5aR	Myeloid	42
CD42a	GPIX	Platelets	23	CD89	FcαR	Myeloid	55-75
CD42b	GPIB, α	Platelets	135, 23	CDw90	Thy-1	Myeloid	25-35
CD42c	GPIB, β	Platelets	22	CD91	α2M-R	Myeloid	600
CD42d	GPV	Platelets	85	CDw92		Myeloid	70
CD44	Pgp-1	Adhesion	80-90	CD93		Myeloid	120
CD44R	Restricted epitope on CD44	Adhesion		CD94	KP43	NK cell	43
CD49a	VLA-1, α1 integrin chain	Adhesion	210	CD95	APO-1, FAS	Activation	42
CD49b	VLA-2, α2 integrin chain	Adhesion	160	CD96	TACTILE	Activation	160
CD49c	VLA-3, α3 integrin chain	Adhesion	125	CD97		Activation	74, 80, 89
CD49d	VLA-4, α4 integrin chain	Adhesion	150, 80, 70	CD98	4F2, 2F3	T cell	80, 40
CD49e	VLA-5, α5 integrin chain	Adhesion	135, 25	CD99	E2, MIC2	T cell	32
CD49f	VLA-6, α6 integrin chain	Adhesion	120, 25	CD99R	CD99 mAb restricted	T cell	32
CD50	ICAM-3	Adhesion	124	CD100	BB18, A8	T cell	150
CD51/CD61	Complex dependent epitope	Adhesion		CDw101	BB27, BA27	T cell	140
CD52	Campath-1	Blind	21-28	CD102	ICAM-2	Adhesion	60
CD62E	E-selectin, ELAM-1	Adhesion	115	CD103	HML-1	Adhesion	150, 25
CD62L	L-selectin, LAM-1, TQ-1	Adhesion	75-80	CD104	β4 integrin chain	Adhesion	220
CD62P	P-selectin, GMP-140, PADGEM	Adhesion	150	CD105	Endoglin	Endothelial	95
CD66a	BGP	Myeloid	180-200	CD106	VCAM-1, INCAM-110	Endothelial	100, 110
CD66b	CD67, p100, CGM6	Myeloid	95-100	CD107a	LAMP-1	Endothelial	110
CD66c	NCA	Myeloid	90-95	CD107b	LAMP-2	Platelet	120
CD66d	CGM1	Myeloid	30	CDw108		Platelet	80
				CDw109	8A3, 7D1	Adhesion	170/150
				CD115	CSF-1R, M-CSFR	Endothelial	150

Table 3.7b *(Continued)*

CD Designation	Common Name	Workshop Section	MW Reduced	CD Designation	Common Name	Workshop Section	MW Reduced
CD66e	CEA, carcinoembryonic antigen	Myeloid	180-200	CDw116	HGM-CSFR, GM-CSFR	Cytokine	75-85
CD67	Now CD66b			CD117	SCFR, cKIT	Cytokine	145
CD70	CD27-ligand	Activation	55, 75, 95, 110, 170	CDw119	IFNγR	Cytokine	90
				CD120a	TNFR; 55kD	Cytokine	55
				CD120b	TNFR; 75kD	Cytokine	75
CDw76	Previously CD76	B cell	NA	CDw121a	IL-1R; Type 1	Cytokine	80
CD79a	mb-1, Igα	B cell	33, 40	CDw121b	IL-1R; Type 2	Cytokine	68
CD79b	B29, Igβ	B cell	33, 40	CD122	IL-2R; 75KD, IL-2Rβ	Cytokine	75
CD80	B7, BB1	B cell	60	CDw124	IL-4R	Cytokine	140
CD81	TAPA-1	B cell	22	CD126	IL-6R	Cytokine	80
CD82	R2, IA4, 4F9	B cell	50-53	CDw127	IL-7R	Cytokine	75
CD83	B Cell	43	CDw128	IL-8R	Cytokine	58-67	
CDw84	B Cell	B cell	73	CDw130	IL-GR-gp130SIG	Cytokine	130

From: Schlossman SF, Boumsell L, Gilks W, et al. CD antigens 1993 (commentary). Blood 1994;83:879–880. Reprinted with permission.

[a] Fifth International Workshop on Human Leukocyte Differentiation Antigens, Boston MA, November 3–7, 1993. Leukocyte Differentiation Antigen Database Version 1.10, July 1994. Available on computer disc. Stephen Shaw, National Institutes of Health.

Table 3.7c
CD Antigens[a]

CD Designation	Common Name/Remarks	Workshop Section	CD Designation	Common Name/Remarks	Workshop Section
CD45RC	Restricted epitope of CD4	Nonlineage	CD141	Thrombomodulin	Endothelial
CD52	CDw52	Nonlineage	C142	Tissue factor	Endothelial
CD65	CDw65	Myeloid	CD143	ACE	Endothelial
CD65s	Sialylated form of CD65	Myeloid	CD144	VE-cadherin	Endothelial
CD66f	PMG-1	Myeloid	CDwj145	Previously inderlined	Endothelial
CD84	CDw84	B cell	CD146	MUC18, S-endo	Endothelial
CD90	CDw90, Thy-1	Adhesion	CD147	Neurothelin, Basigin	Endothelial
CD101	CDw101	Myeloid	CD148	HPTP eta, p260 phosphatase	Nonlineage
CD109	CDw109	Endothelial	CDw149	MEM-133	Nonlineage
CD114	G-CSFR	Myeloid	CDw150	SLAM, IPO-3	Nonlineage
CD116	CDw116, GM-CSFR	Cytokine	CD151	PETA-3	Platelet
CD121a	CDw121a, IL-IR; type 1	Cytokine	CD152	CTLA-4	T cell
CDw123	IL-3Rα	Cytokine	CD153	CD30L	T cell
CD124	CDw124, IL-4R	Cytokine	CD154	CD40L, T-BAM	T cell
CDw125	IL-5Rα	Cytokine	CD155	PVR	Myeloid
CD127	CDw127, IL-7R	Cytokine	CD156	ADAM8. MS2 (mouse homologue)	Myeloid
CD130	CDw130, IL-6R-gp130 signal transducer	Cytokine	CD157	BST-1, M0-5	Myeloid
CDw131	Common β	Cytokine	CD158a	p58.1, MHC class 1-specific NK receptors	NK cell
CD132	Common γ	Cytokine			
CD134	OX40	Cytokine	CD158b	p58.2, MHC class 1-	NK cell

(Continued)

Table 3.7c (Continued)

CD Designation	Common Name/Remarks	Workshop Section	CD Designation	Common Name/Remarks	Workshop Section
				specific NK receptors	
CD135	Flt3, Flk2	Cytokine	CD161	NKRP-1	NK cell
CDw136	MSP-R	Cytokine	CD162	PSGL-1	Adhesion
CDw137	4-1BB	Cytokine	CD163	M130	Myeloid
CD138	Syndecan-1	B cell	CD164	MGC-24	Adhesion
CD139	Previously undefined	B cell	CD165	GP37/AD2	Adhesion
CD140a	PDGFrα	Endothelial	CD166	ALCAM	Adhesion
CD140b	PDGFrβ	Endothelial			

Abbreviations: ACE, angiotensin-converting enzyme; ALCAM, activated leukocyte cell adhesion molecule; CD30L, CD30 ligand; G-CSFR, granulocyte colony-stimulating factor receptor; GM-CSFR, granulocyte-macrophage colony-stimulating factor receptor; IL, interleukin; MHC, major histocompatibility complex; MSP-R, macrophage-stimulating protein receptor; NK, natural killer; NKRP1, NK receptor P1; PDGFR, platelet-derived growth factor receptor; PSGL-1, P-selectin glycoprotein ligand 1; PVR, polio virus receptor; VE, vascular endothelial.

[a] From Sixth International Workshop on Human Antigens, Kobe, Japan, November 10–14, 1996. Immunology Today 1997;18:100–101.

BIBLIOGRAPHY

Articles

Abruzzo LV, Jaffe ES, Cotelingam JD, et al. T-cell lymphoblastic lymphoma with eosinophilia associated with subsequent myeloid malignancy. Am J Surg Pathol 1992;16(3):236–245.

Adriaansen HJ, te Boekhorst PA, Hagemeijer AM, et al. Acute myeloid leukemia M4 with bone marrow eosinophilia (M4Eo) and inv(16) (p13q22) exhibits a specific immunophenotype with CD2 expression. Blood 1993;81:3043–3051.

Baumann I, Nenninger R, Harms H, et al. Image analysis detects lineage-specific morphologic markers in leukemic blast cells. Am J Clin Pathol 1996;105(1):23–30.

Bitter MA, Neilly ME, LeBeau MM, et al. Rearrangements of chromosome 3 involving bands 3q21 and 3q26 are associated with normal or elevated platelet counts in acute nonlymphocytic leukemia. Blood 1985;66:1362–1370.

Buccheri V, Shetty V, Yoshida N, et al. The role of an anti-myeloperoxidase antibody in the diagnosis and classification of acute leukemia: a comparison with light and electron microscopy cytochemistry. Br J Haematol 1992;80:62–68.

Cerezo L, Shuster LL, Pullen DJ, et al. Laboratory correlates and prognostic significance of granular acute lymphoblastic leukemia in children: a Pediatric Oncology Group Study. Am J Clin Pathol 1991;95:526–531.

Crisan D. Molecular diagnostic testing for determination of myeloid lineage in acute leukemias. Ann Clin Lab Sci 1994;24(4):355–363.

Crisan D, Kaplan S, Penchansky L, et al. A new procedure for cell lineage determination in acute leukemias. Myeloperoxidase mRNA detection. Diagn Mol Pathol 1993;2(2):65–73.

Cuneo A, Kerim S, Vanderberghe E, et al. Translocation t(6;9) occurring in acute myelofibrosis, myelodysplastic syndromes, and acute nonlymphocytic leukemia suggests multipotent stem cell involvement. Cancer Genet Cytogenet 1989;42:209–219.

Davey FR, Abraham N, Brunetto VL, et al. Morphologic characteristics of erythroleukemia (acute myeloid leukemia); FAB M6: a CALGB study. Am J Hematol 1995;49:29–38.

Del Poeta G, Stasi R, Venditti A, et al. CD7 expression in acute myeloid leukemia. Leuk Lymphoma 1995;17:111–119.

Del Poeta G, Stasi R, Venditti A, et al. Prognostic value of cell markers in de novo acute myeloid leukemia. Leukemia 1994;8:388–394.

DeRossi G, Grossi C, Foa R, et al. Immunophenotype of acute lymphoblastic leukemia cells: the experience of the Italian Cooperative Group (Gimema). Leuk Lymphoma 1993;9:221–228.

Erber WN, Asbahr H, Rule SA, et al. Unique immunophenotype of acute promyelocytic leukaemia as defined by CD9 and CD68 antibodies. Br J Haematol 1994;88:101–104.

Hammer RD, Collins RD, Ebrahimi S, et al. Rapid immunocytochemical analysis of acute leukemias. Am J Clin Pathol 1992;97(6):876–84.

Harada H, Ason H, Kyo T, et al. A specific chromosome abnormality of t(4;12) (q11–12;p13) in CD7+ acute leukemia. Br J Haematol 1995;90:850–854.

Hatta Y, Iwata T, Takeuchi J, et al. Complete remission in a patient with hypoplastic acute lymphoblastic leukemia induced by granulocyte-colony-stimulating factor. Acta Haematologica 1995;94:39–43.

Invernizzi R, Rosanda C, Basso G, et al. Granular acute lymphoblastic leukemia in children. Haematologica 1992;77:30–34.

Ishikawa K, Seriu T, Watanabe A, et al. Detection of neoplastic clone in hypoplastic and recovery phases preceding acute lymphoblastic leukemia by in vitro amplification of rearranged T-cell receptor delta chain gene. J Pediatr Hematol Oncol 1995;17:270–275.

Kawai S, Zha Z, Yamamoto Y, et al. Clinical significance of childhood acute myeloid leukemias expressing lymphoid-associated antigens. Pediatr Hematol Oncol 1995;12:463–469.

Kornblau SM, Thall P, Huh YO, et al. Analysis of CD7 expression in acute myelogenous leukemia: martingale residual plots combined with optimal cutpoint analysis reveals absence of prognostic significance. Leukemia 1995;9:1735–1741.

Kovarik P, Shrit MA, Yuen B, et al. Hand mirror variant of adult acute lymphoblastic leukemia. Evidence for a mixed leukemia. Am J Clin Pathol 1992;98:526–530.

Lauria F, Raspadori D, Ventura MA, et al. The presence of lymphoid-associated antigens in adult acute myeloid leukemia is devoid of prognostic relevance. Stem Cells 1995;13:428–434.

Loken MR, Shah VO, Datillio KL, et al. Flow cytometric analysis of human bone marrow. Normal erythroid development. Blood 1987;62:722–728.

Macedo A, Orfao A, Gonzalez M, et al. Immunological detection of blast cell subpopulations in acute myeloblastic leukemia at diagnosis: implications for minimal residual disease studies. Leukemia 1995;9(6):993–998.

Maynadie M, Bailly F, Casasnovas RO, et al. Immunophenotype in erythroleukemia secondary to myelodysplastic syndrome (letter). Blood 1992;80:1097.

Pui CH, Raimondi SC, Head DR, et al. Characterization of childhood acute leukemia with multiple myeloid and lymphoid markers at diagnosis and at relapse. Blood 1991;78:1327–1337.

Raimondi R, Pellizzari G, Rodeghiero F. Single step immunophenotyping of acute leukemias not classifiable by standard morphology and cytochemistry: a practical approach. Haematologica 1993;78(6 Suppl 2):66–72.

Reinhertz EL, Kung PC, Goldstein G, et al. Discrete stages of human intrathymic differentiation: analysis of normal thymocytes and leukemic lymphoblasts of T-cell lineage. Proc Natl Acad Sci USA 1980;77:1588–1592.

Robertson MJ, Cochran KJ, Cameron C, et al. Characterization of a cell line, NKL, derived from an aggressive human natural killer cell leukemia. Exper Hematol 1996;24:406–415.

San Miguel JF, Gonzalez M, Canizo MC, et al. Surface marker analysis in acute myeloid leukemia and correlation with FAB classification. Br J Haematol 1986;64:547–560.

Scott AA, Head DR, Kopecky KJ, et al. HLA-DR–, CD33+, CD56+, CD16– myeloid/natural killer cell acute leukemia: a previously unrecognized form of acute leukemia potentially misdiagnosed as French-American-British acute myeloid leukemia M3. Blood 1994;84:244–255.

Soni M, Brody J, Allen SL, et al. Immunophenotypic changes between diagnosis and relapse in childhood acute lymphoblastic leukemia. Leukemia 1995;9(9):1523–1533.

Urbano-Ispizua A, Matutes E, Villamor N, et al. The value of detecting surface and cytoplasmic antigens in acute myeloid leukemia. Br J Haematol 1992;81:178–183.

Wiernik P. Translocation (2;9) (p12;p23) in a case of acute leukemia with t(4;11)(q21;q23). Lack of rearrangement of the kappa and interferon gene loci. Cancer Genet Cytogenet 1992;60:82–85.

Zucker ML, Plapp FV, Rachel JM, et al. An adult case of acute biphenotypic leukemia with characteristic mixed morphology. Mo Med 1993;99:601–604.

Review Articles

Campana D, Hansen-Hagge T, Matutes E, et al. Phenotypic, genotypic, cytochemical, and ultrastructural characterization of acute undifferentiated leukemia. Leukemia 1990;4:620–624.

Catovsky D, Matutes E, Buccheri V, et al. A classification of acute leukemia for the 1990s. Acta Haematol 1991;62:16–21.

Foon KA, Todd RF II. Immunologic classification of leukemia and lymphoma. Blood 1986;68:1–31.

Hogan TF, Koss W, Murgo AJ, et al. Acute lymphoblastic leukemia with chromosomal 5;14 translocation and hypereosinophilia: case report and literature review. J Clin Oncol 1987;5(3):382–390.

Hurwitz CA, Mirro J. Mixed-lineage leukemia and asynchronous antigen expression. Hematol Oncol Clin North Am 1990;4:767–794.

Matutes E, Catovsky D. The value of scoring systems for the diagnosis of biphenotypic leukemia and mature B-cell disorders. Leuk Lymphoma 1994;13(Suppl 1):11–14.

Pui CH. Acute leukemias with the t(4;11) (q21;q23). Leuk Lymphoma 1992;7:173–179.

Schumacher HR, Cotelingam JD. Hypereosinophilic syndrome terminating in monocytic leukemia (AML-5a): case 6. In: Chronic leukemia: approach to diagnosis. New York: Igaku-Shoin, 1993:245–249.

Taylor CG, Stasi R, Bastianelli C, et al. Diagnosis and classification of the acute leukemias: recent advances and controversial issues. Hematopathol Mol Hematol 1996;10:1–38.

Wibowo A, Pankowsky D, Mikhael A, et al. Adult acute leukemia: hand mirror cell variant. Hematopathol Mol Hematol 1996;10:85–89.

CHAPTER 4

Cytogenetics

GENERAL COMMENTS

Cytogenetic studies provide important information that is clinically relevant for diagnosis and prognosis of human malignancies. It has become increasingly clear that an acquired genetic alteration underlies most, if not all, malignancies and that the genetic abnormality is usually discernible at the level of the chromosome. Since nonrandom chromosomal abnormalities have been so closely associated with distinct types of acute leukemia, their recognition can allow a diagnosis independent of other criteria. This led to the formation of the Morphology, Immunology, and Cytogenetics (MIC) Cooperative Study Group that based diagnosis on the findings in these three areas. Furthermore, the insight that cytogenetic information provides regarding the identification and localization of genes involved in malignant transformation is a major contribution of cytogenetic analysis; however, conventional karyotypic analysis has limitations in that only a few cells arrested in metaphase are analyzed. Also, analysis is entirely dependent on production of high-quality metaphase preparations, and it is not possible to perform on cells that are terminally differentiated since such cells never enter mitosis. In addition, conventional cytogenetic analysis also is significantly restricted for cells that have low mitotic rates or cannot easily be grown in culture. Finally, conventional cytogenetic analysis is limited because it is labor intensive, requires highly trained technologists for interpretation, and is greatly time consuming. For some of these reasons, fluorescent in situ hybridization (FISH) has been developed to overcome the inherent disadvantages in routine cytogenetics. This will be discussed below.

Although specific cytogenetic abnormalities in acute lymphoblastic leukemia (ALL) can be related to immunophenotype, with the exception of t(8;14)(q24;q32) and its FAB L3 variants, they do not show a close relationship to the FAB subtype. Contrariwise, in acute myeloid leukemia (AML), chromosomal abnormalities including t(8;21)(q22;q22) FAB M2;t(15;17) FAB M3; or inv (16) (p13;q22) FAB M4Eo have been associated with specific morphologic features. Table 4.1 shows nonrandom chromosomal aberration, frequency, disease characteristics, and prognosis in some of the more important acute leukemias.

Recently, in situ hybridization (ISH) techniques have been developed to complement routine cytogenetics. ISH is based on the property of single-stranded DNA to hybridize specifically with complimentary sequences. It can be used to visualize whole chromosomes (chromosome painting) or specific multiple or single copy DNA sequences present on chromosomes. The procedure involves DNA probes of known specificity that are labeled with ^{3}H or, preferably, with nonisotopic haptens such as biotin or digoxigenin.

Table 4.1

Examples of Nonrandom Cytogenetic Abnormalities Associated With Specific Types of Acute Myelocytic and Lymphoblastic Leukemia

Chromosome Aberration	Frequency[a]	Disease[b] Characteristics	Prognosis (Median Survival)
Acute Myelocytic Leukemia (AML)			
t(8;21)(q22;q22) and variants	~12%	M2, Auer rods Rarely M4	Fair to good
t(15;17)(q22;q21)	~10% (>90% of APL)	M3, also microgranular form, DIC	Fair to good
inv(16)(p13q22)/t(16;16)	~10% (>25% of M4)	M4 "eo"; abnormal eosinophils in bone marrow Recurrence as chloroma in CNS	Good
t(9;11)(q22;q23)	5% to 6%	M5	Poor
t(11q23)	>70% secondary leukemia[c]	M4 to M5	Poor
t(6;9)(p23q34)	~1%	M2, M4, MDS Basophilia in bone marrow	Poor
t(8;16)(p11;p13)	<1%	M5 with phagocytosis	Undetermined
inv (3)(q21q26),t(3;3)	3% to 5%	M4, other AML with dysmegakaryopoiesis, thrombocytosis	Undetermined
t(1;3)(p36;q21)			
t(1;22)(p13;q13)	<1%	M7	Undetermined
t(1;7)(q10;p10)	1%	Secondary AML	Poor
t(3;21)(q26;q22)	<1%	Secondary AML	Poor
Numerical abnorm:			
+4, +11, +21	1% to 3%	M4, M1 to M7	Undetermined
+8, −5, −7	>40%	All FAB types, secondary AML and MDS	Poor to very poor
Deletions:			
5q, 7q, 12p, 20q	>40%	All FAB types, secondary AML and MDS	Poor to very poor
Acute Lymphoblastic Leukemia (ALL)			
Hyperdiploid (>50)	30% (childhood)	Common ALL	Good to very good
	~15% (adult)	Low WBC	Fair to good
Hyperdiploid (47–50)	7% to 8% (childhood)		Fair

Table 4.1 (Continued)

Chromosome Aberration	Frequency[a]	Disease[b] Characteristics	Prognosis (Median Survival)
Pseudodiploid	40% (childhood)	Bulky disease	Poor to very poor
(See translocations)	>50% (adult)	Phenotype corresponding to specific translocation	
Diploid	10% to 30%	T-All (30%)	Fair to poor
Hypodiploid	7% to 8%		Fair to poor
Near haploid	<1%		Poor
t(9;22)(q34;q11)	1% to 3% (childhood)	Precursor B	Very poor
	>30% (adult)		
t(4;11)(q21;q23)	>50% (infancy)	Early pre B, biphenotypic, high WBC	Very poor
	~2% (adult)		(8 months)
t(1;19)(q23;p13)	5% to 6% (childhood)	Pre-B, high WBC	Fair to poor
t(8;14)(q24;q32),t(2;8) and (8;22)	~3% to 4%	B-ALL (L3), high WBC	Very poor
		CNS leukemia, abdominal tumors	
t(11;14)(p13;q11)	1%	T-ALL (7%)	Poor
t(10;14)(q24;q11)	1%	T-ALL (5% to 10%)	Poor
t(8;14)(q24;q11)	<1%	T-ALL (2%)	Poor
t(1;14)(p32;q11)	<1%	T-ALL (3%)	Poor
del 6q/abn 6q	~10%	No specificity	Undetermined
del /abn 9p21-22	~10%	High risk features	Poor
abn 12p	~10%	B-lineage >1 T-ALL	Variable
dic (9;12)(p11;p12)	Rare	B-progenitor	Good

From: Hagemeijer A, Grosveld G. Molecular cytogenetics of leukemia. In: Henderson ES, Lister TA, Greaves MF, eds. Leukemia. 6th ed. Philadelphia: WB Saunders, 1996:133.

[a] Frequency in % of total number of cytogenetically abnormal cases in AML and ALL.
[b] Acute leukemia classification according to the French, American, British (FAB) classification.
[c] Secondary myeloid leukemia in patients treated with inhibitors of DNA-topoisomerase II.

CNS, central nervous system; DIC, disseminated intravascular coagulation; MDS, myelodysplastic syndrome; WBC, white blood cell count.

Subsequently, probes and target DNA present in the chromosomes of interphase cells and metaphases are denatured and hybridized together at high stringency. The hybridized probes are visualized by immunodetection using antibodies marked by fluorochromes (FITC, Texas red), enzymes, or by autoradiography in the case of radioactive labeling. FISH has proven to be the most practical and straightforward technique for both routine and research applications. Furthermore, the combined use of multiple probes and multiple colors makes it possible to investigate multiple or complex genetic questions in a single experiment. FISH bridges the gap in resolution between cytogenetics and molecular DNA techniques and is becoming increasingly sensitive. Some examples of molecular cytogenetic applications are presented in Table 4.2.

The advantage of interphase cytogenetics is that it allows the analysis of all cells, not just the few arrested in metaphase. Hundreds or even thousands of cells can easily be studied, in comparison with 20 or so cells that are te-

Table 4.2
Examples of Molecular Cytogenetic Applications in the Study of Leukemia

Probes	Target Cells	Results	Sensitivity	Combination With Other techniques
Chromosome-specific DNA repeats	Metaphase and interphase cells	Numeric abnormalities	Trisomy: high Monosomy: good	+++ +++
Chromosome/bands[a] paints	Metaphases	Marker identification	Good	+[b]
Marker paints	Control metaphases	Marker identification	Good	+[b]
Ph paints	Leukemic metaphases	Ph detection	Good	+[b]
YACS cosmid/phage	Metaphase and interphase cells	Structural aber- ration		
		Variant trans- location	High	+++
		Specific trans- location	High	+++
Unique sequences	Metaphases and interphase[c] DNA halo	Gene mapping and gene rearrangement	Variable	+++

From: Hagemeijer A, Grosveld G. Molecular cytogenetics of leukemia. In: Henderson ES, Lister TA, Greaves MF, eds. Leukemia. Philadelphia, WB Saunders, 1996:135.

[a] For example, cloning or amplification of chromosomes obtained by flow sorting and bands obtained by microdissection.
[b] Limiting factor is the possibility of applying combined identification of cells in metaphases.
[c] Multicolor ISH of neighboring sequences.

diously analyzed conventionally. The analysis of large numbers of cells is significant because it permits the detection of low-frequency abnormalities that are otherwise difficult to detect. Also, specimens that would not be suitable for culturing and conventional techniques could still yield useful cytogenetic data. In addition, such analysis has application in studying cells from tumors with low proliferative activity or from tumors that are difficult to maintain in short-term cultures. Finally, interphase analysis is easily learned and does not require special training for interpretation, and it allows some correlation of cytogenetic findings with morphology. The latter is not possible with the routine cytogenetic study because all nuclear detail is lost in metaphase.

FISH and whole chromosome painting have been used to advantage in chronic myelogenous leukemia (CML), t(9;22); trisomy and tetrasomy 8, FAB M3, t(15;17); monosomy 7; trisomy 21; B cell ALL t(1;19); FAB M2, t(8;21); FAB M4Eo, [inv (16)] to mention a few in the recent literature. Image analysis has been used by some to analyze this data. Also, some investigators have begun to attempt to analyze large numbers of FISH-labelled cells by flow cytometry. Undoubtedly, this will have future value in detecting minimal residual disease.

ACUTE UNDIFFERENTIATED LEUKEMIA (AUL)

For the most part, past cytogenetic studies on AUL were inaccurate due to lack of sophisticated diagnostic techniques. With the introduction of new techniques such as two, three, and four color fluorescence analysis by combined flow cytometry, FISH, numerous specific monoclonal antibodies, and ultrastructural studies, many previously classified cases of AUL have been described as new entities, i.e., FAB M0, megakaryoblastic leukemia, and biphenotypic leukemia. In the future, with DNA rearrangement and MPEX gene studies, AUL should become a rarity. For example, in 1989 Ludwig et al. studied a series of 35 cases of acute leukemia in children (less than 1 year old) previously classified as ALL or AUL. They found 17 cases of ALL, 17 of mixed lineage leukemia, and only 1 case without criteria for classification, i.e., AUL. Interestingly, Moore and Andreef reported AUL in association with t(4;11) (q21;q23), a karyotypic abnormality with higher prevalence in infants and young children characterized by an undifferentiated hematopoietic precursor cell. In addition to this cytogenetic relationship to AUL, the United Kingdom Cancer Cytogenetics Group analyzed 73 patients of acquired, single autosomal trisomies associated with hematological disorders, excluding trisomy 8 cases in myeloid conditions and trisomy 12 in lymphoid conditions. Of the 73 patients, 60 had myeloid disorders, 12 had lymphoid disorders, and 1 case was an AUL. The AUL demonstrated a single trisomy 11 clone.

Table 4.3
Summary of Cytogenetic Findings

Diagnosis FAB Subtype	Cytogenetics	Comment	Reference
AUL	t(4;11)(q21;q23) trisomy 11 (single case report)	Fewer cases will be reported as technology advances	Medical Onc. A comprehensive review. Pazdur R, ed. PRR, NY: 1993:11 Leuk Res 1992;16:841–851
Hypocellular/ aplastic ALL	No distinctive cytogenetic characteristics	Hypocellular/aplastic phase followed by overt leukemia in weeks or few months	Atlas tumor pathol. Tumors of the bone marrow. Fascicle 9, Washington AFIP, 1993:115
Granular ALL	Variable: some children with Down's syndrome, others Ph[1]	Prognosis poor response in adults; prognosis controversial in children	Am J Clin Pathol 1983; 79:426–430 Haematologica 1992;77: 30–34 Am J Clin Pathol 1991; 95:526–531
ALL with eosinophilia	t(5;14)(q31;q32)	Eosinophilia due to release of IL3 by leukemic lymphoblasts. Eosinophils lack cytogenetic abnormality	Blood 1990;76:285–289 Med Pediatr Onc 1984; 12:33–37
ALL t(4;11)	t(4;11)(q21;q23)	Morphology FAB ALL L1, L2; FAB AML 5a; bilineage biphenotypic, AUL. Topoisomerase II inhibitors seem to involve band 11q23	Blood 1994;83:2274–2284 Ann Hematol 1992;65: 143–146
ALL-hand mirror cell variant	Variable cytogenetic findings	Heterogeneous group of disorders. Some may be mixed leukemias with adhesion molecules	Am J Clin Pathol 1992; 98:526–530 Hematopathol Molec Hematol 1996;10:85–98
ANKCL	Complex variable abnormalities	Subgroups of LGL Leukemias appear to demonstrate cytogenetic variability	Cancer 1995;75:2472–2483 Exp Hematol 1996;24: 406–415
AML M0	-5/5q- OR -7/7q- commonly seen complex karyotypes	Cytogenetics frequently similar to therapy related AML. Cytogenetic groups may be associated with characteristic clinicobiologic features. Chromosome rearrangements may account for poor outcome.	Blood 1995;85:3688–3694 Ann Hematol 1996;74: 208–215 Blood 1994;83: 1619–1625

(Continued)

Table 4.3 *(Continued)*

Diagnosis FAB Subtype	Cytogenetics	Comment	Reference
AML M6	Frequent involvement of chromosomes 5 and 7. Evidence suggests three or more karyotypic abnormalities are associated with increased pro-erythroblasts and poor prognosis	Erythroleukemia is a hetero-geneous disorder. Those with myeloblasts (Di Guglielmo's syndrome). Those with proerythroblasts (Di Guglielmo's disease). Needs clarification of criteria for diagnosis	Am J Clin Pathol 1992;98: 34–40 Br J Haematol 1990;75:346–354 Am J Hematol 1995;49:29–38
Acute basophilic leukemia	t(6;9)(p23;q34) seen in AML M2 baso, M1, M2, MDS	Heterogeneous disorder with Philadelphia chromosome most likely a CML variant. ABL needs further evaluation	Cancer Genet Cytogenet 1995;84:99–104 Am J Clin Pathol 1991;96: 160–170 Am J Hematol 1989;31: 133–135
Eosinophilic leukemia/hyper-eosinophilic syndrome	No specific chromosomal abnormality. Multiple chromosomal aberrations reported	Heterogeneous disorder needs clarification	Br J Haematol 1987;67: 25–31 Leukemia 1988;2 394–397. Br J Haematol 1986;62:659–669
Hypocellular/ Aplastic AML	5q-, monosomy 7, trisomy 8. Normal sometimes progress to MDS or leukemia	Hypocellular/aplastic non-leukemic cases require care-ful monitoring for evolu-tionary change	Blood 1991;77:1397–1398 Exp Hematol 1987;15: 1134–1139
CD7 AML	Variable from normal to complex karyotypes	Heterogeneous disorder or technical problems with diagnosis	Cancer Genet Cytogenet 1996;86:31–34 Cancer Genet Cytogenet 1994;73:69–74
AML inv 3(q21;q26)	High levels of *EVI*-1 transcripts in RNA. No increase thrombopoietin	Increased platelets and mega-karyocytes not related to gene abnormality in region of thrombopoietin gene	Br J Haematol 1995;91: 425–427 Blood 1994;84:2681–2688
NK-myeloid leukemia	Most cases normal karyo-types. Few with abnorm-alities of 17q	Important to distinguish such cases from FAB AML M3, 3v since NK-myeloid leukemias do not respond to ATRA	Blood 1994;84:244–255
Billineage/ biphenotypic acute leukemia	Karyotypes frequently associated with mixed leukemias t(9;22); 11q23, trisomy 13; 14q32	Multipotent stem cell in-volved in mixed leukemia. Lineage switch occurs more frequently in children, leukemias T-cell subtype switch to AML, 11q23 abnormalities fre-quently noted	Blood 1990;76:150–156 Leukemia 1995;9:1305–1312 Am J Clin Pathol 1992;98: 526–530

ACUTE LYMPHOBLASTIC LEUKEMIA (ALL)

Hypocellular/Aplastic ALL

Acute leukemia presenting as aplastic anemia may be indistinguishable from true aplastic anemia in the early stages. Such a presentation is more common in childhood, particularly with ALL. A transient recovery of normal blood counts is frequently noted after corticosteroid treatment. Nevertheless, ALL commonly occurs within 6 months of the onset of aplasia. There are no distinctive morphologic, immunophenotypic, or cytogenetic characteristics associated with the overt leukemic phase. Nevertheless, chromosomal abnormalities would support a leukemic process rather than an aplastic disorder, especially if they are known leukemic karyotypes.

Granular ALL

Granular ALL is usually of B-cell precursor common immunophenotype. No consistent cytogenetic associations have been reported, but several cases have been seen in children with Down syndrome, and others have been associated with the Philadelphia chromosome. Some authors reported with karyotypes 47, XX, +21, t(12;17); 46/60 both chromosome lines unanalyzable; 46,XX/46,XX,22q−/48,XX,22q−,+22q−,+? marker and other unidentifiable changes (Philadelphia chromosome positive); 46,XX(normal); 46/90 (both clones unanalyzable). Although this variant may represent an entity with poor response to therapy in adults, the prognosis in children has been controversial with some authors considering the finding unimportant, whereas others have suggested it portends a worse prognosis.

ALL with eosinophilia

Mild to marked eosinophilia is occasionally noted at diagnosis. In some cases the eosinophilia is so pronounced that the diagnosis of ALL was obscured. Some of these cases have been confused with a myeloproliferative disorder. Others have clinical manifestations of the hypereosinophilic syndrome (HES). Tono-oka et al. reported a case of an 8-year-old boy with HES associated with acute lymphoblastic leukemia FAB L1. He had an eosinophilia of 120×10^9/L with few lymphoblasts. Bone marrow examination revealed many mature eosinophils and 20% lymphoblasts. Direct chromosome analysis of the bone marrow cells revealed that 12.5% of the spontaneously dividing cells had an abnormal karyotype of 46XY, t(5;14)(q31;q32). Meeker et al. have successfully cloned the t(5;14)(q31;q32) from two B-lineage acute lymphocytic leukemias with eosinophilia. In both cases, this translocation joined the IgH gene and the interleukin 3 (IL3) gene. In one patient, excess IL3 messenger ribonucleic acid (mRNA) was produced by the leukemic cells. In the other, serum IL3 levels were measured and shown to correlate with disease activity. There was no evidence of excess granulocyte-macrophage colony-stimulating factor (GM-CSF) or IL5 expression. They suggested that ALL with eosinophilia in these cases may arise in part because of the t(5;14) that activates the IL3 gene. Therefore, the eosinophilia is thought to be reactive and the result of excessive IL3 release. This is further supported by the finding that eosinophils in this disorder lack the cytogenetic abnormality.

ALL t(4;11)

The t(4;11)(q21;23) has been associated with FAB ALL L1, L2 morphology of an early B-precursor phenotype, with FAB AML M5a, with bilineage-biphenotypic leukemia, and with AUL (Fig. 4.1). This translocation has a high prevalence in infants and young children, and all seem to have a poor outcome. There has been great interest recently concerning

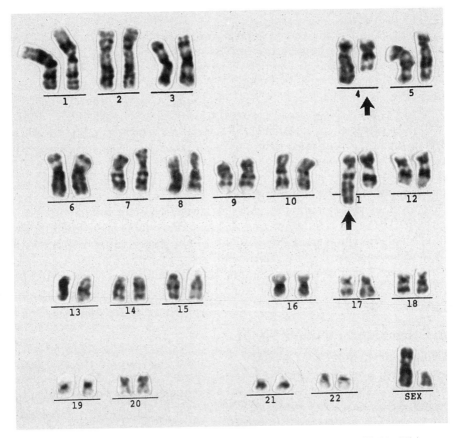

Figure 4.1. Karyotype of a trypsin banded metaphase illustrating the t(4;ll)(q21;q23) in a patient with ALL L2 morphology and a biphenotypic acute leukemia. The rearranged chromosomes 4 and 11 are identified with arrows. Courtesy of Linda Shepard.

t(4;11)(q21;q23) because of the demonstration of the involvement of ALL1 locus on band 11q23 and of the AF4 locus. The presence of heptameric and nonameric sequences close to the breakpoints suggests that a mistake of the recombinase system physiologically active in pro-B elements may be responsible for the translocation. Heerema et al. observed that patients with the t(4;11) showed shorter disease-free survival than patients demonstrating only the 11q23 breakpoint suggesting that the specific translocation, and not the breakpoint per se, may be associated with the poor prognosis of these infants. Auxenfants et al. reported two cases of secondary ALL with t(4;11)(q21;q23) and reviewed seven previously published cases. They noted that most patients had received a combination of topoisomerase II inhibitors (antracyclines, mitoxantrone, or the epipodophyllotoxin derivatives VP16 or VM26) and cyclophosphamide that have been implicated in the pathogenesis of secondary AML with 11q23 rearrangements. Such observations suggest that the 11q23 region of the genome could be particularly susceptible to chemical agents.

Zhang et al. studied three patients with secondary acute leukemia after treatment with topoisomerase II inhibitor agents by means of FISH and combined immunophenotyping and FISH (FICTION). Two patients had FAB AML 5a; one had pre-B-acute leukemia. The 11q23 rearrangements were detected in all cases. They were due to translocations t(11;19) (q23;p13.3), t(11;16)(q23;p13), and t(4;11)(q21;q23), respectively. FISH with yeast artificial chromosome *(YAC) PROBE 13HH4* spanning the *ALL-1* gene on 11q23 confirmed that in each case the ALL-1 gene had been disrupted by the translocations. This study further confirms the relationship between secondary acute leukemias with 11q23 rearrangements and previous chemotherapy with topoisomerase II inhibitor agents. It also illustrates that myeloid and lymphoid leukemias have a common biological background. The authors substantiated this hypothesis by means of combining immunophenotyping and FISH (FICTION) by showing that both the FAB M5a cells and pro-B-ALL cells with ALL-1 rearrangement expressed CD34. Such a finding suggests that the cell of origin of secondary AML and ALL with 11q23 rearrangement is an immature hematopoietic progenitor cell.

ALL-Hand Mirror Variant (HMV)

Cytogenetic studies on ALL-HMV have been quite varied. Normal karyotypes have been reported in a number of cases. Stern et al. reported an ALL-HMV of T cell origin that showed a bimodal chromosome number of 49 (49, XX, +10, −21, +3 rings) and a high degree of polyploid modal karyotype with 94 chromosomes (6 no. 10, 3 no. 18, 2 no. 21 chromosomes, 3 ring chromosomes, plus 4 copies of each other chromosome). The patient was mentally retarded and had a constitutional chromosomal abnormality 46, XX, with a ring 21. Kovarik et al. reported a case of ALL-HMCV by morphology that on analysis was a biphenotypic (mixed) leukemia. Interestingly, the cytogenetic studies demonstrated a recurring abnormality involving 11q23, specifically the t(11;19)(q23;p13.1). The t(11;19) has been observed in biphenotypic leukemias as well as T-cell acute lymphoblastic leukemia.

Kao et al. have reported a trisomy 4 in a case of acute undifferentiated myeloblastic leukemia with hand mirror cells (HMCs). Also, Sun and Weiss published a case of HMV in a microgranular acute promyelocytic leukemia with t(15;17).

Therefore, cytogenetic findings are varied in leukemic patients with HMCs, supporting the heterogeneous nature of the occurrence of these cells in leukemia. To date, subgroups appear to exist, i.e., null cell ALLs resistant to treatment, mixed leukemias, those with adhesion molecules; all of which need further investigation for better classification so appropriate therapy can be instituted.

AGGRESSIVE NK CELL LEUKEMIA (ANKCL)

Cytogenetic studies in the large granular lymphocytic (LGL) leukemias (T-LGL, NK-LGL) have not shown consistent clonal abnormalities, suggesting that they represent a heterogeneous group of disorders. Robertson et al. have studied an ANKCL cell line and determined the karyotype to be 47, XY, add (1)(q42), +6 del (6)(q15q23), del (17)(p11). These cells expressed CD2, CD6, CD11a, CD26, CD27, CD29, CD38, CD43, CD58, CD81, CD94, CD95, class II MHC, and the C1.7.1. They did not express detectable levels of CD3, CD4, CD5, CD8, CD14, CD19, CD20, CD28, alpha/beta or gamma/delta T cell receptors on the cell surface. The NK cell line was capable of mediating antibody-dependent cellular cytotoxicity, as well as natural killing. Brody et al. studied an acute agranular CD4 positive NK cell leukemia with an abnormal karyotype (44XY, 5q−, −13, 13q+, −15). The immunophenotype was CD3−, CD56+, CD4+, CD8−, CD15+, TCR1−, and TCR2−, with germline immunoglobulin and T-cell receptor genes. Studies for genomic EBV or HHV-6 revealed no abnormalities. These findings support heterogeneity of cytogenetic, and immunophenotypic findings in subgroups of the LGL leukemias.

ACUTE MYELOID LEUKEMIA (AML)

AML M0

FAB AML M0 very frequently carries cytogenetic abnormalities common to MDS or secondary AML, such as −5/5q− or −7/7q− deletions and/or complex karyotypes (Fig. 4.2). Cuneo et al. performed cytogenetic studies on 26 patients with de novo FAB AML M0. They found clonal abnormalities in 21 cases (80.7%); 12 of which had a complex karyotype. Partial or total monosomy 5q and/or 7q was found, either as the sole aberration or in all

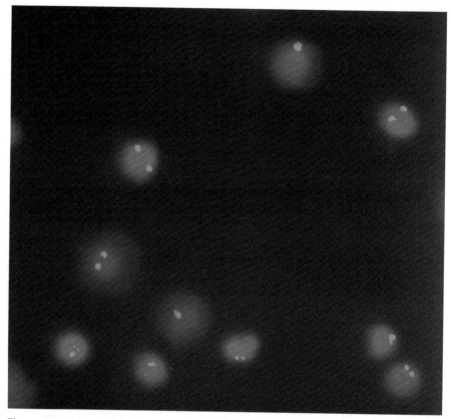

Figure 4.2. Metaphase demonstrating FISH with the probe labelled with FITC for chromo-some 7 in a patient with AML M0. Note cells with one signal confirming the absence of one chromosome 7. Courtesy of Ruth Blough.

abnormal metaphases, in 11 patients; in 8 cases, additional chromosome changes were present, including rearrangements involving 12p12-13 and 2p12-15 seen in three cases each. Five patients had trisomy 13 as a possible primary chromosome change; in five cases, nonrecurrent chromosome abnormalities were observed. Comparison of these features with chromosome data from 42 patients with FAB AML M1 showed that abnormal karyotypes, complex karyotypes, unbalanced chromosome changes ($-5/5q-$ and/or $-7/7q-$ and $+13$) were observed much more frequently in FAB AML M0 than in FAB AML M1. Patients with abnormalities of chromosome 5 and/or 7 frequently showed trilineage myelodysplasia and low white blood cell count. Despite their relatively young age, complete remission was achieved in 4 of 11 patients only. Elderly males with $+13$ had frequent professional exposure to myelotoxic agents. Cuneo et al. concluded that FAB AML M0 shows a distinct cytogenetic profile, partially recalling that of therapy-related AML; different cytogenetic groups exist that show characteristic clinicobiologic features; and chromosome rearrangements may partially account for the unfavorable outcome. Amadori et al. found similar cytogenetic results and noted that the FAB AML M0 was very often associated with the minimal drug resistant (MDR) phenotype. Stasi et al. observed the most common findings were trisomy 8 and aberrations of chromosome 7 in 13 cases they evaluated.

Some authors have applied FISH in two cases of FAB AML M0 with a reciprocal translocation t(12;13)(p13;q14) to investigate the position of the *RB* gene with respect to the breakpoint at 13q14. The results showed that the *RB* gene was proximal to the breakpoint and apparently not split in either case.

AML M6-Erythroleukemia

The FAB criteria for erythroleukemia is restricted in that only those cases with myeloblastic elements are classified as erythroleukemia (Di Guglielmo's syndrome). There is, however, another form of erythroleukemia, variously referred to as Di Guglielmo's disease, pure erythroleukemia, erythremic myelosis, or M6b, in which the predominant immature elements are proerythroblasts. Some authors have noted increased karyotypic abnormalities in this pure erythroleukemia population (Di Guglielmo's disease) that was associated with a shorter survival time.

Kowal-Vern et al. performed chromosomal analysis on 8 of 23 patients with erythroleukemia. Two patients had a normal karyotype and five had chromosome 5 and/or 7 aberrations. There does not appear to be a distinction between therapy-related and *de novo* erythroleukemia because both have abnormal chromosomes 5 and 7. Cuneo et al. attempted to classify subsets with erythroleukemia on the basis of cytogenetic findings. They determined that the subset with the higher percentage of proerythroblasts/basophilic erythroblasts (pure erythroleukemia M6b) had a higher incidence of more than two karyotypic abnormalities and a shorter survival. Contrariwise, the subset with fewer immature erythroid cells (greater erythroid maturation potential) had either normal or only one or two karyotypic abnormalities and a longer survival time (myeloblastic component, M6a). Also, Bernheim et al. noted increased karyotypic abnormalities with an excess of proerythroblasts.

Finally, in cytogenetic analysis of 27 cases of erythroleukemia, Davey et al. found 14 (52%) with karyotypic abnormalities. Five (19%) were simple (less than 3 karyotypic abnormalities), while 9 (33%) were complex (greater than or equal to 3 abnormalities). Complete or partial loss of 5, 7, or 12p, or the presence of trisomy 8 were noted in 11 of 27 (41%) of their patients. They concluded that the morphology of the erythroblasts may correlate with cytogenetic abnormalities and rate of complete remission.

Diagnostic criteria need to be clarified in the erythroleukemias. Many of the current cases are being placed in a category of the myelodysplastic syndromes. Prognosis and appropriate therapy are not possible until such diagnostic criteria, which should include cytogenetic data, are established.

Acute Basophilic Leukemia (ABL)

The cytogenetic findings in ABL are varied; most likely due to the heterogeneity of this rare disorder and lack of clear diagnostic criteria.

Shah et al. reported a case of ABL in a 61-year-old black woman with 85 to 90% basophils in the peripheral blood and bone marrow. This resulted as a transformation from essential thrombocythemia. There was a cytogenetic change from 46XX karyotype to 46XX 2p+ in 66 to 90% of cells in the bone marrow during the transformation.

Kubota et al. observed a 20-month-old child with AML and basophilic differentiation. The leukemic cells had a cytogenetic abnormality of t(9;11)(p22;q23). Although immature blasts responded well to induction therapy with etoposide, the leukemic cells that were more differentiated toward basophils were quite refractory to the drug.

Peterson et al. described eight cases of ABL. In six of the eight cases, basophilic involvement was not apparent by light microscopy. Cytogenetic analysis revealed the cases were heterogeneous. Three had a Philadelphia chromosome, suggesting they were really CML with basophilic expression. Interestingly, none showed t(6;9).

Shekkter-Levin et al. reported a case of Kostmann disease in a 12-year-old child in which cytogenetic analysis of the bone marrow cells revealed an abnormal clone with monosomy 7 and trisomy 21. Monosomy 7 was also confirmed by FISH. After 2 months of follow up, the patient presented with ABL, expressing the same bone marrow chromosome abnormalities as before.

Perhaps more clearly defined cases that seem to represent a variant are those designated AML M2 baso. This variant is characterized by granulocytic maturation and a variable infiltrate of blast cells with basophilic granules, and is associated with t(6;9)(p23;q34). The involved genes have been cloned and named DEK (on chromosome 6) and CAN (on chromosome 9). Besides AML M2 baso, this translocation may be present in AML M1, M4, MDS (Fig. 4.3), and acute myelofibrosis. Although the detection of basophilic precursors may be frequent, it is not a constant finding in Giemsa-stained preparations. Also, it has been observed that patients with apparently de novo AML and t(6;9) display multilineage myelodysplasia. Such data suggest that t(6;9) may represent a nonselective cytogenetic marker associated with a group of neoplasias deriving from a myeloid stem cell. Also, basophilia in AML has been reported with abnormalities of the short arm of chromosome 12.

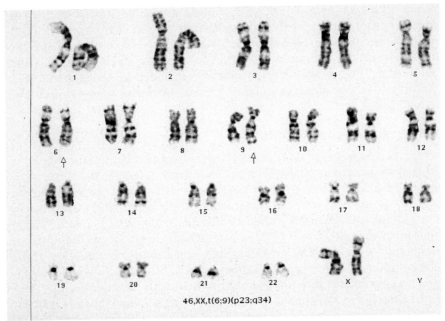

46,XX,t(6;9)(p23;q34)

Figure 4.3. Karyotype of a trypsin-Giemsa banded metaphase cell showing the t(6;9)(p23;q34) in a patient with RAEB. The rearranged chromosomes are identified by arrows. Courtesy of Margie Hayes and Howard Saal.

Eosinophilic Leukemia (EL)/Hypereosinophilic Syndrome (HES)

Cytogenetic analysis becomes extremely important when attempting to distinguish between EL and HES. Fauci et al. proposed empirical criteria for diagnosing HES and identified three groups of patients with different clinical courses: (1) asymptomatic cases with a favorable course; (2) symptomatic patients with organ involvement and a more serious prognosis; (3) patients with hepatosplenomegaly, cytogenetic abnormalities, blastic crisis evolution, and features that are consistent with an aggressive leukemia.

The diagnosis of EL continues to remain a problem. Both acute and chronic forms have been observed. This compounds the problem because large numbers of immature elements have not been present in many cases and the putative blasts have not been fully characterized. Moreover, the association of HES and other entities have frequently detracted against the existence of EL in pure form. Furthermore, although a variety of chromosomal abnormalities, including Ph[1] chromosome trisomy 7, 8, 9, and 10, 9q−, translocation abnormalities of 12p13, +(10;11), t(5;11), t(8;21), a short Y chromosome, and isochromosome 17 have been observed and catalogued by Keene et al. No specific marker appears to be present; however, they have demonstrated translocation abnormalities of chromosome 12p13 in cases of acute EL, Ph[1] negative myeloproliferative disease, and ALL. They speculate that a gene regulating eosinophil production may be located at this site, which is in proximity to the oncogene c-*Ki RAS* 2. The only well-documented case of acute secondary EL is reported by Maeda et al., that developed 8 years after melphalan treatment for multiple myeloma in a 71-year-old woman. The cytogenetic abnormalities included a 5q− and monosomy 7, similar to those observed in other patients with treatment induced AML (t-AML).

Hypocellular/Aplastic AML

Cytogenetic analysis of bone marrow that is hypocellular/aplastic may be extremely important in determining the underlying diagnosis and correct therapeutic course. Applebaum et al. suggested that a clonal cytogenetic abnormality in aplastic anemia is an indication that the disorder is a myelodysplastic syndrome. They studied 183 patients with aplastic anemia and noted that only seven (4%) showed clonal chromosomal abnormalities frequently seen in MDS or AML, including deletion of the long arm of chromosome 5, monosomy 7, and trisomy 8. Although five patients (3%) had no cytogenetic abnormalities and subsequently developed either MDS or leukemia, they concluded that all patients with aplastic anemia may have some risk of developing leukemia. They further suggested, however, that those with a cytogenetic abnormality are at especially high risk. By contrast Moormeier et al. observed three patients with hypocellular marrow, mild dysplasia, and trisomy 6 who did not have the clinical characteristics of MDS or AML. Also, two of the three patients responded to treatment directed at autoimmune mediated aplastic anemia. These findings suggest that clonal cytogenetic abnormalities may not always be a specific indicator of MDS or AML. Nevertheless, the finding of an abnormality common to MDS and AML, such as −5, del(5q2), −7, del (7q) and trisomy 8, would support a premalignant myeloid proliferation. This is supported by the report of Horsman et al., who identified an unusual pediatric patient among 12 patients with myelodysplasia and unbalanced translocation involving chromosomes 1 and 7: −7, +del(1), +(1;7)(p11;p11). The 16-year-old male patient developed myelodysplasia and evolving acute leukemia, which were preceded by a 7-year history of marrow hypoplasia. The remaining patients were adults with clinical and hematologic findings similar to other reported cases with this chromosomal abnormality. The late appearance of this unbalanced clonal abnormality in this patient with marrow hypoplasia documents the importance of close cytogenetic follow up of all patients with suspected bone marrow injury. Furthermore, some investigators have observed cases in which an aplastic bone marrow evolved to a cellular dysplastic marrow and terminated as frank AML. These cases require careful monitoring of peripheral blood, bone marrow, cytogenetics, and molecular genetics to determine the subtle changes that underlie such an evolutionary process.

CD7 Positive AML

CD7 is expressed in 10 to 30% of AML patients usually with FAB M0, M1, and M5a and immature markers such as CD34, TdT, and HLA-DR. There are controversial reports in the literature regarding the prognostic value of CD7 expression in AML. Also, cytogenetic analysis has varied from normal karyotypes to complex karyotypes. Shimamoto et al. evaluated six patients with AML expressing CD7+. Five patients demonstrated FAB AML M1 morphology and one FAB AML M2. Cytogenetic analysis demonstrated normal karyotypes in all cases. On the contrary, Secco et al. reported six patients with acute leukemia characterized by the presence of a t(10;11)(p11-15;q13-q23), either as the sole cytogenetic abnormality or as part of a complex abnormal karyotype. Four patients were CD7+ AMLs; two with morphological features of FAB AML M5a and two with FAB ALL L1 morphological features. The two FAB AML M5as revealed the following karyotypes: 46, XY, t(10;11)(p11.2;q23) and 46, XY, t(10;11)(p12;q13). The FAB ALL L1 revealed more complex karyotypes: 47, XX, t(10;11)(p15;q21), +19 and 54, XY, dup(1) (p22.3p36), +1, +6, +7, t(10;11)(p13;q21), del (13)(q13q22) X2, +13, +19, +20,+21, +mar. The patient with FAB AML M5a morphology and (p11.2;q23) was evaluated by serial phenotypic studies during the course of the disease. Interestingly, a switch from monocytic to lymphoid morphology at the time of the first or second relapse was observed. This paralleled the appearance of a pre-T ALL immunophenotype with co-expression of the myeloid antigen CD33. These phenotypic changes occurred without apparent alteration in the genotype since t(10;11)(p11.2;q23) remained the only cytogenetic aberration at all stages of the disease. The authors speculate that their findings suggest that the t(10;11) variant of 11q aberrations occurs in a bipotential myelomono-cytic/T-lymphoid stem cell. In support of abnormal complex karyotypes in CD7+ AML, Del Poeta et al. have most recently reported an article on CD7 expression in AML.

From the wide variation in the results of karyotypic analysis and treatment response, either the CD7+ AMLs represent a broad heterogeneous group of disorders, or diagnostic techniques need more careful scrutiny.

AML inv 3(q21;q26)

Structural alterations occur in the long arm of chromosome 3 in approximately 2% of patients with AML or MDS. The major alterations are inv 3(q21;26) and t(3;3)(q21;q26) and are often classified as the 3(q21;q26) syndrome. Patients with these abnormalities have normal platelet counts or thrombocytosis that can exceed 1000 × 10⁹/L. AMLs with these abnormalities are difficult to classify morphologically. They have been classified as FAB AML M1, M4, and M6. Patients with these aberrant karyotypes have an unfavorable prognosis and generally have associated abnormalities of megakaryocytopoiesis, including increased megakaryocytes and micromegakaryocytes. Bouscary et al. studied the thrombopoietin gene which maps to human chromosome 3q26. Although the *EVI*-1 gene maps to this region 3q26:q27 and high levels of transcripts could be detected in mRNA in four patients with typical 3(q21:q26) syndrome, no thrombopoietin transcripts were detectable by reverse transcriptase polymerase chain reaction (RT-PCR) technique on the same mRNA samples. These results demonstrate that the thrombopoietin gene transcription is not activated in patients with 3q26 chromosomal abnormality and that abnormal thrombopoietin production is not responsible for the observed thrombocytosis.

Myeloid/NK-Leukemia

NK-myeloid leukemia has been a previously unrecognized form of acute leukemia that is remarkably similar to acute promyelocytic leukemia; especially the microgranular variant (FAB AML M3v). Scott et al. evaluated 350 cases of de novo AML and identified 20 cases (6%) with a unique immunophenotype CD33+, CD56+(NK), CD11a+, CD13^{dim}, CD15^{dim}, CD34+/-, HLA-DR-, CD16-. Multicolored flow cytometric assays confirmed the coexpression of myeloid (CD33, CD13, CD15) and NK cell associated (CD56) antigens in each case. All 20 cases lacked the t(15;17) and 17 cases tested lacked the promyelocytic/retinoic acid receptor alpha (RAR alpha) fusion transcript in RT-PCR assays. Cytogenetic analysis revealed that 12 cases had normal karyotypes, whereas two cases had abnormalities of chromosome 17q1 with del (17)(q25) and another had t(11;17)(q23;q21) and the promyelocytic leukemia zinc finger/RAR alpha fusion transcript. All cases tested (6/20) failed to differentiate in vitro in response to all-trans-retinoic acid (ATRA), suggesting that these cases may account for some acute promyelocytic leukemias that have not shown a clinical response to ATRA. Recognition of these NK-myeloid leukemias should be important in distinguishing those ATRA-nonresponsive cases from ATRA-responsive true acute promyelocytic leukemias. Both cytogenetic analysis and appropriate immunophenotyping play an important pivotal role in establishing the correct diagnosis.

BILINEAGE/BIPHENOTYPIC ACUTE LEUKEMIA

Cytogenetic analysis has allowed investigators to recognize karyotypes that are more frequently associated with biphenotypic leukemias. The karyotypes include t(9;22)(q34, q11) (Fig. 4.4); aberrations of chromosome 11 at band q23 e.g. t(4;11)(q21;q23), del (11)(q23); and of chromosome 14 at band q32, and trisomy 13. Rare cases of mixed leukemia have been reported with trisomy 4 and t(7;12). The demonstration of these cytogenetic entities lends support to the belief that biphenotypic and bilineal acute leukemias involve a multipotent stem cell and an early maturation arrest.

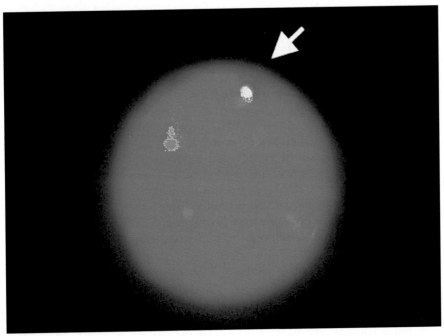

Figure 4.4. Detection of the *BCR-ABL* fusion genes in interphase in an ALL with a Ph¹ chromosome. After hybridization, the *ABL* probe was detected with Texas red and the BCR probe with FITC (green). The locations of the normal copies of *BCR* and *ABL* in the nuclei are indicated by the isolated red and green signals. The *BCR-ABL* fusion gene produces closely spaced red and green signals, sometimes appearing yellow (arrow). Courtesy of Ruth Blough.

Hirsch-Ginsberg et al. studied five patients with Ph¹+ acute leukemia by means of ultrastructural, phenotypic, and molecular analysis. Four of the five patients had acute mixed lineage leukemia (AMLL). One patient had acute unclassifiable leukemia. Of the four patients classified as AMLL, three showed myeloid and lymphoid features, with one showing myeloid, T cell, and B cell features. The last case exhibited T cell and B cell features only. The authors concluded that such studies support the concept of phenotypic and molecular heterogeneity in Ph¹+ acute leukemia, and support the use of lineage-associated molecular probes to define lineage at an earlier stage than previously possible.

Mirro et al. evaluated seven cases of acute leukemia associated with t(4;11)(q21;q23). Serial analysis of karyotype, immunophenotype, and heavy-chain immunoglobulin genes revealed changes in these biological markers over time, suggesting continued chromosomal rearrangement and gene modulation after the leukemogenic event in those patients with t(4;11)(q21;q23). They concluded that acute leukemia with the t(4;11)(q21;q23) abnormality has mixed lineage characteristics as a result of leukemogenesis in a multipotential progenitor cell or aberrant gene expression later in differentiation. The critical aberration apparently resides on chromosome 11 at band q23 since other cases have been recorded with this abnormality. Interestingly, Kovarik et al. reported a biphenotypic leukemia with t(11;19)(q23[1] 3.1) with HMCs. They suggested that patients with acute leukemia-HMV be evaluated for AMLL. Guilhot et al. evaluated 16 cases of t(11;19) acute leukemia and reviewed the literature. They described four hematological groups: (1) B-lineage ALL, (2) biphenotypic leukemia, (3) T-ALL, (4) AML M4 or M5. The biphenotypic leukemias were most often CD19+ ALL, but demonstrated expression of differentiation markers of monocytic lineage. The B lineage and biphenotypic leukemias were predominantly found in female infants. Recently, Domer et al. have reported rearrangements of the *MLL* (mixed lineage leukemia) gene in the human 11q23 cytogenetic locus in acute leukemia patients who have received topoisomerase II inhibitors for previous neoplasms. Such therapy-related acute leukemias are associated with poor response to therapy and unfavorable outcomes.

Although a 14q32 abnormality is associated with t(14;18)(q32;q21) in 75% of follicular and 30% of diffuse lymphomas of B cell origin, Hayashi et al. reported a 14q32 translocation in 10 children of 440 cases of newly diagnosed ALL and AML. Remarkably, mixed-lineage expression was found in 6 of these 10 cases, but in only 21 of the other 430 cases. Thus, in addition to the well described 11q23 translocations and t(9;22), 14q32 translocations appear to be associated with mixed lineage antigen expression.

Barr and Bloomfield reported on trisomy 13 in acute leukemia. They noted that this karyotypic abnormality is seen primarily in older males and has been associated with treatment-associated acute leukemia, acute leukemia evolved from MDS, and in de novo leukemia. Immunophenotyping studies have shown an undifferentiated phenotype or biphenotypic markers in most cases. Some have been classified as AMLL. Patients with trisomy 13 have a low complete remission rate, brief remission duration, and unfavorable outcome.

Lineage switch is an expression of markers of one lineage at diagnosis, but markers of a different phenotype or lineage at the time of leukemia relapse. The switch, which is more frequent in children with T-cell subtype, usually occurs following a treatment interval of 1 year or more from the time of the initial diagnosis. Most cases have involved a lineage switch from ALL to AML. Although cytogenetic studies have revealed involvement of chromosome 11, region 11q23 as the most common structural abnormality, lineage switch has occurred in Ph+ acute lymphoblastic leukemia (FAB ALL L1 to FAB AML M2), and t(5;14) (q33-34;q11) (ALL to AML).

FISH and whole chromosome painting have been used to advantage in a case of FAB AML M2 where chromosome 11 was rearranged in a highly complex manner, involving band 11q23. Routine G banding failed to identify this complex rearrangement. Also, FISH has been used to advantage in an AMLL case with unbalanced 7;12.

BIBLIOGRAPHY

Articles

Abdelaal AF, Silver RT, Macera MJ, et al. Characterization of chromosome 11 with a complex inversion and deletion in an AML [M2] using fluorescence in situ hybridization. Acta Haematologica 1995;94:152–155.

Anastasi J, Feng J, Dickstein JI, et al. Lineage involvement by BCR/ABL in Ph+ lymphoblastic leukemias: chronic myelogenous leukemia presenting in lymphoid blast vs Ph+ acute lymphoblastic leukemia. Leukemia 1996;10(5):795–802.

Anonymous. Primary, single, autosomal trisomies associated with haematological disorders. United Kingdom Cancer Cytogenetics Group (UKCCG). Leukemia Research 1992;16(9):841–851.

Appelbaum FR, Barroll J, Storb R, et al. Clonal cytogenetic abnormalities in patients with otherwise typical aplastic anemia. Exp Hematol 1987;15:1134–1139.

Bernell P, Jacobsson B, Nordgren A, et al. Clonal cell lineage involvement in myelodysplastic syndromes studied by fluorescence in situ hybridization and morphology. Leukemia 1996;10(4):662–668.

Bernheim A, Berger R, Daniel MT, et al. Malignant and reactive erythroblasts in erythroleukemia (M6). Cancer Genet Cytogenet 1983;10:1–10.

Bernheim A, Duverger A, Fouquet F, et al. FISH diagnosis of t(8;21) in a myelodysplasia secondary to Hodgkins lymphoma. Leukemia 1995;9(1):107–108.

Bouscary D, Fontenay-Roupie M, Chretien S, et al. Thrombopoietin is not responsible for the thrombocytosis observed in patients with acute myeloid leukemias and the 3q21q26 syndrome. Br J Haematol 1995;91(2):425–427.

Brody JP, Allen S, Schulman P, et al. Acute agranular CD4-positive natural killer cell leukemia. Comprehensive clinicopathologic studies including virologic and in vitro culture with inducing agents. Cancer 1995;75(10):2474–2483.

Cerezo L, Shuster JJ, Pullen DJ, et al. Laboratory correlates and prognostic significance of granular acute lymphoblastic leukemia in children. A Pediatric Oncology Group study. Am J Clin Pathol 1991;95:526–531.

Cuneo A, Ferrant A, Michaux JL, et al. Cytogenetic profile of minimally differentiated (FAB M0) acute myeloid leukemia: correlation with clinicobiologic findings. Blood 1995;85(12):3688–3694.

Cuneo A, Van Orshoven A, Michaux JL, et al. Morphologic, immunologic, and cytogenetic studies in erythroleukemia: evidence for multilineage involvement and identification of two distinct cytogenetic-clinicopathologic types. Br J Haematol 1990;75:346–354.

Davey FR, Abraham N Jr, Brunetto VL, et al. Morphologic characteristics of erythroleukemia (acute myeloid leukemia; FAB-M6): a CALGB study. Am J Hematol 1995;49(1):29–38.

DeLaat CA, Files B, Harris RE, et al. Undifferentiated acute leukemia and lineage infidelity (difficulties in classification and management). Med Pediatr Oncol 1990;18(1):15–21.

Del Poeta G, Stasi R, Venditti A, et al. CD7 expression in acute myeloid leukemia. Leuk Lymphoma 1995;17:111–119.

Domer PH, Head DR, Renganathan N, et al. Molecular analysis of 13 cases of MLL/11q23 secondary acute leukemia and identification of topoisomerase II consensus-binding sequences near the chromosomal breakpoint of a secondary leukemia with the t(4;11). Leukemia 1995;9:1305–1312.

Filatov LV, Behm FG, Pui CH, et al. Childhood acute lymphoblastic leukemia with equivocal chromosome markers of the t(1;19) translocation. Genes Chromosom Cancer 1995;13(2):99–103.

Fradera J, Velez-Garcia E, White JG. Acute lymphoblastic leukemia with unusual cytoplasmic granulation: a morphologic, cytochemical and ultrastructural study. Blood 1986;68:406–411.

Hay CR, Barnett D, James V, et al. Granular common acute lymphoblastic leukemia in adults: a morphologic study. Eur J Haematol 1987;39:299–305.

Hayashi Y, Pui CH, Behm FG, et al. 14q32 translocations are associated with mixed-lineage expression in childhood acute leukemia. Blood 1990;76(1):150–156.

Heerema NA, Arthur DC, Sather H, et al. Cytogenetic features of infants less than 12 months of age at diagnosis of acute lymphoblastic leukemia: impact of the 11q23 breakpoint on outcome: a report of the Children's Cancer Group. Blood 1994;83(8):2274–2284.

Hirsch-Ginsberg C, Childs C, Chang KS, et al. Phenotypic and molecular heterogeneity in Philadelphia chromosome-positive acute leukemia. Blood 1988;71(1):186–195.

Horsman DE, Massing BG, Chan KW, et al. Unbalanced translocation (1;7) in childhood myelodysplasia. Am J Hematol 1988;27(3):174–178.

Invernizzi R, Rosanda C, Basso G, et al. Granular acute lymphoblastic leukemia in children. Haematologica 1992;77:30–34.

Johansson B, Arheden K, Hoglund M, et al. Fluorescence in situ hybridization analysis of whole-arm 7;12 translocations in hematologic malignancies. Genes Chromosom Cancer 1995;14(1):56–62.

Kao YS, McCormack C, Vial R. Trisomy 4 in a case of acute undifferentiated myeloblastic leukemia with hand mirror cells. Cancer Genet Cytogenet 1990;45:265–268.

Kovarik P, Shrit MA, Yuen B, et al. Hand mirror variant of adult acute lymphoblastic leukemia. Evidence for a mixed leukemia. Amer J Clin Pathol 1992;98(5):526–530.

Kowal-Vern A, Cotelingam J, Schumacher HR. The prognostic significance of proerythroblasts in acute erythroleukemia. Am J Clin Pathol 1992;98:34–40.

Kubota M, Akiyama Y, Tabata Y, et al. Acute nonlymphocytic leukemia with basophilic differentiation and t(9,11)(p22,q23) in a child. Am J Hematol 1989;31(2):133–135.

Lai M, Hamasaki K, Tokioka M, et al. A case of hand mirror cell variant of acute lymphoblastic leukemia. Acta Med Okayama 1980;34(4):283–287.

Ludwig WD, Bartram CR, Harbott J, et al. Phenotype and genotype heterogeneity in infant acute leukemia. Acute lymphoblastic leukemia. Leukemia 1989;3:431–439.

Maeda K, Van Slyck E, Van Dyke D. Multiple myeloma terminating in acute eosinophilic leukemia. Cancer Genet Cytogenet 1985;16:81–89.

Martinez-Climent JA, Thirman MJ, Espinosa R, et al. Detection of 11q23/MLL rearrangements in infant leukemias with fluorescence in situ hybridization and molecular analysis. Leukemia 1995;9(8):1299–1304.

Maschek H, Kaloutsi V, Rodriquez-Kaiser M, et al. Hypoplastic myelodysplastic syndrome: incidence, morphology, cytogenetics, and prognosis. Ann Hematol 1993;66(3):117–122.

Meeker TC, Hardy D, Willman C, et al. Activation of the interleukin-3 gene by chromosome translocation in acute lymphocytic leukemia with eosinophilia. Blood 1990;76(2):285–289.

Mirro J, Kitchingman G, Williams D, et al. Clinical and laboratory characteristics of acute leukemia with the 4;11 translocation. Blood 1986;67(3):689–697.

Moormeier JA, Rubin CM, Le Beau MM, et al. Trisomy 6: a recurring cytogenetic abnormality associated with marrow hypoplasia. Blood 1991;77:1397–1398.

Muhlematter D, Castagne C, Bruzzese O, et al. Tetrasomy 8 in a patient with acute nonlymphocytic leukemia: a metaphase and interphase study with fluorescence in situ hybridization. Cancer Genet Cytogenet 1996;89(1):44–48.

Murakawa M, Shibuya T, Taniguchi S, et al. Acute eosinophilic leukemia in a patient with preexistent myelodysplastic syndrome. Acta Haematologica 1991;86(1):42–45.

Parreira L, Tavares de Castro J, Hibbin JA, et al. Chromosome and cell culture studies in eosinophilic leukaemia. Br J Haematol 1986;62(4):659–669.

Peterson LC, Parkin JL, Arthur DC, et al. Acute basophilic leukemia. A clinical, morphologic, and cytogenetic study of eight cases. Am J Clin Pathol 1991;96(2):160–170.

Reardon DA, Handson CA, Roth MS, et al. Lineach switch in Philadelphia chromosome-positive acute lymphoblastic leukemia. Cancer 1994;73(5):1526–1532.

Robertson MJ, Cochran KJ, Cameron C, et al. Characterization of a cell line, NKL, derived from an aggressive human natural killer cell leukemia. Exp Hematol 1996;24(3):406–415.

Scott AA, Head DR, Kopecky KJ, et al. HLA-DR−, CD33+, CD56+, CD16− myeloid/natural killer cell acute leukemia: a previously unrecognized form of acute leukemia potentially misdiagnosed as French-American-British acute myeloid leukemia-M3. Blood 1994;84(1):244–255.

Scott AA, Head DR, Kopecky KJ, et al. Acute leukemia with t(10;11)(p11-p15;q13-q23). Cancer Genet Cytogenet 1996;86(1):31–34.

Secco C. Killer cell leukemia. Experimental Hematology 1996;24:406–415.

Shah I, Lewkow LM, Koppitch F. Acute basophilic leukemia. Am J Med 1984;76(6):1097–1099.

Shah-Reddy I, Mirchandani I, Bishop CR. Hand mirror cell leukemia—immunologic and ultrastructural studies. Cancer 1981;47(4):715–719.

Shekhter-Levin S, Penchansky L, Wollman MR, et al. An abnormal clone with monosomy 7 and trisomy 21 in the bone marrow of a child with congenital agranulocytosis (Kostmann disease) treated with granulocyte colony-stimulating factor. Evolution towards myelodysplastic syndrome and acute basophilic leukemia. Cancer Genet Cytogenet 1995;84(2):99–104.

Stasi R, Del Poeta G, Venditti A, et al. Analysis of treatment failure in patients with minimally differentiated acute myeloid leukemia (AML-M0). Blood 1994;83(6):1619–1625.

Stein P, Peiper S, Butler D, et al. Granular acute lymphoblastic leukemia. Am J Clin Pathol 1983;79(4):426–430.

Stern R, Widirstky ST, Wurster-Hill DH, et al. Hand-mirror cell leukemia associated with mental retardation: immunologic, chromosome, and morphological studies. Blood 1979;54(3):703–712.

Sun T, Weiss R. Hand mirror variant of microgranular acute promyelocytic leukemia. Leukemia 1991;5(3):266–269.

Suzukawa K, Parganas E, Gajjar A, et al. Identification of a breakpoint cluster region 3' of the ribophorin I gene at 3q21 associated with the transcriptional activation of the EVII gene in acute myelogenous leukemias with inv(3) (q21q26). Blood 1994;84(8):2681–2688.

Tono-oka T, Sato Y, Matsumoto T, et al. Hypereosinophilic syndrome in acute lymphoblastic leukemia with a chromosome translocation [t(5q;14q)]. Med Ped Oncol 1984;12(1):33–37.

Tosi S, Stilgenbauer S, Giudici G, et al. Reciprocal translocation t(12;13)(p13;q14) in acute nonlymphoblastic leukemia: report and cytogenetic analysis of two cases. Cancer Genet Cytogenet 1994;77(2):106–110.

Whitlock JA, Raimondi SC, Harbott J, et al. t(5;14)(q33-34;q11), a new recurring cytogenetic abnormality in childhood acute leukemia. Leukemia 1994;8(9):1539–1543.

Wibowo A, Pankowsky D, Mikhael A, et al. Adult acute leukemia: hand mirror cell variant. Hematopathol Molec Hematol 1996;10:85–98.

Zhang Y, Poetsch M, Weber-Matthiesen K, et al. Secondary acute leukaemias with 11q23 rearrangement: clinical, cytogenetic, FISH and FICTION studies. Br J Haematol 1996;92(3):673–680.

Review Articles

Amadori S, Venditti A, Del Poeta G, et al. Minimally differentiated acute myeloid leukemia (AML-M0): a distinct clinicobiologic entity with poor prognosis. Ann Hematol 1996;72(4):208–215.

Anastasi J. Interphase cytogenetic analysis in the diagnosis and study of neoplastic disorders. Am J Clin Pathol 1991;95(Suppl 1):522–528.

Auxenfants E, Morel P, Lai JL, et al. Secondary acute lymphoblastic leukemia with t (4;11): report on two cases and review of the literature. Ann Hematol 1992;65(3):143–146.

Baer MR, Bloomfield CD. Trisomy 13 in acute leukemia. Leuk Lymphoma 1992;7(1-2):1–6.

Bentz M, Dohner H, Cabot G, et al. Fluorescence in situ hybridization in leukemias: "the fish are spawning." Leukemia 1994;8(9):1447–1452.

Fauci AS, Harley JB, Roberts WC, et al. The idiopathic hypereosinophilic syndrome. Ann Intern Med 1982;97:78–92.

Fox JL, Hsu PH, Legator MS, et al. Fluorescence in situ hybridization: powerful molecular tool for cancer prognosis. Clin Chemistry 1995;41(11):1554–1559.

Hagemeijer A, Grosveld G. Molecular cytogenetics of leukemia. In: Henderson ES, Lister TA, Greaves MF, eds. Leukemia. Philadelphia: WB Saunders, 1996:131–144.

Huret JL, Brizard A, Slater R, et al. Cytogenetic heterogeneity in t(11;19) acute leukemia: clinical, hematological and cytogenetic analyses of 48 patients—updated published cases and 16 new observations. Leukemia 1993;7(2):152–160.

Keene P, Mendelow R, Pinto MR, et al. Abnormalities of chromosome 12p13 and malignant proliferation of eosinophils: a nonrandom association. Br J Haematol 1987;67:25–31.

Moore DF, Andreef MA. The acute leukemias. In: Pazdur R, ed. Medical oncology: a comprehensive review. Huntington, NY: PRR, 1993:5–28.

Nichols CR, Breeden ES, Loehrer PJ, et al. Secondary leukemia associated with a conventional dose of etoposide: review of serial germ cell tumor protocols. J Nat Cancer Inst 1993;85(1):36–40.

Shimamoto T, Ohyashiki JH, Ohyashiki K, et al. Clinical and biologic characteristics of CD7+ acute myeloid leukemia. Our experience and literature review. Cancer Genet Cytogenet 1994;73(1):69–74.

CHAPTER 5

Molecular Genetics

GENERAL COMMENTS

The relative importance of traditional techniques used in the diagnosis of hematological malignancies has altered during the past decade. Morphology, cytochemistry, and histology continue to maintain a central role, but the importance of cytochemistry has declined, except in the diagnosis of acute myeloid leukemia (AML). This has been largely due to the impact of immunohistochemistry and immunophenotyping. Immunophenotyping is of major importance in the diagnosis of acute lymphoblastic leukemia (ALL), some categories of AML, and the lymphoproliferative disorders. Cytogenetic analysis is an essential part of the cornerstone of diagnosis of the acute leukemias along with morphology, cytochemistry, immunohistochemistry, and immunophenotyping.

Although molecular genetics was born in the 1980s and intense application of this technology has occurred concerning the leukemias and other hematological malignancies resulting in great insights into the biology and understanding of leukemogenesis, the practical use of this discipline in the diagnosis and classification of the acute leukemias has been limited. The reasons for this are multifold. Firstly, immunoglobulin heavy-chain (IgH) and T-cell receptor (TCR) gene rearrangements are nonspecific findings in acute leukemia and cannot help to correctly characterize undifferentiated blasts. Secondly, specific molecular rearrangements are typical rearrangements of chromosomal translocations that, in most cases, can be determined by conventional cytogenetic analysis. Also, DNA probes are frequently not available because of failure to accurately identify the gene sequencing or, once recognized, the breakpoints may be variable or multiple. Finally, and perhaps the most important in the current health care atmosphere is cost. This must be weighed in regard to benefit to the patient's care. Will the test make a difference in a treatment decision, in outcome, in patient comfort?

Nevertheless, it is becoming more apparent that information generated from molecular analysis can be important information that impacts on diagnosis, patient care, and treatment decisions. For example, routine karyotypic analysis has rarely detected the cryptic t(12;21)(p12-13;q22) leading to *TEL/AML 1* fusion in childhood ALL. Recently, this gene fusion has been recognized as the most frequent genetic rearrangement in childhood ALL. Evidently, this finding is worldwide since using the reverse transcriptase polymerase chain reaction (RT-PCR) assay has demonstrated a 17% frequency of this translocation in the ALL population overall and 19% in patients with B-lineage ALL, similar to previous findings in Caucasian children in France and the United States. These findings have important significance since conventional cytogenetic analysis frequently fails to identify the translocation; and, of greater consequence, fails to identify the t(12;21) positive ALL subgroup of patients who do not require intensive treatment for cure. In addition, the detection of chimeric *BCR-ABL*, and *PBX1-E2A* genes in ALL is crucial for identifying subsets with a biologic and clinical specificity. Similarly the *AML-1/ETO* and the *PML-RARA* fusion genes can be detected with greater sensitivity and alacrity by polymerase chain reaction (PCR) than conventional cytogenetic analysis in patients with FAB AML M2 and AML M3, respectively (Fig. 5.1). As noted with t(12;21), it has become increasingly clear that some leukemias have biologically relevant molecular defects in the absence of a karyotypic abnormality. Also, apparently uniform chromosomal abnormalities such as t(9;22), t(8;14), t(1;19), or t(15;17) may differ at the molecular level, possibly with clinical repercussions. Finally, other defects such as the SIL-TAL 1 recombination on 1p32 or the *SET-CAN* rearrangement on 9p34 can only be recognized at a molecular level because they affect a submicroscopic chromosomal region. Pertinent to our understanding of molecular genetics is our comprehension of the mechanisms of oncogenesis that are shown in Figure 5.2. Note that three general mechanisms are involved in oncogenesis: (1) fusion of proto-oncogenes to form oncogenes, (2) mutation of proto-oncogenes, and (3) loss of tumor-suppressing ability. The latter can also occur in the leukemias. Table 5.1 lists the unusual and controversial leukemias in regard to molecular diagnosis.

Since the observation that chromosomal alterations of human neoplasms are nonrandom, conventional karyotyping of banded chromosomes played an important role in diagnosis, prognosis and management of patients. This technique suffers from inherent limitations. Conventional karyotyping requires viable dividing cells that can be arrested in metaphase. In addition, cells with low mitotic activity, terminally differentiated cells and specimens with a large number of normal cells are suboptimal for conventional karyotyping.

During the last decade, fluorescent in situ hybridization (FISH) identifies chromosomal alteration of interphase (nonmitotic cells). This technique can be easily applied to cases not suitable for Southern blot analysis and, more importantly, can detect chromosomal abnormalities in cases where conventional cytogenetic studies are normal and the diagnosis based on cell morphology is debatable.

Molecular techniques require the availability of deoxyribonucleic acid (DNA) probes specific for the chromosomal aberrations seen in leukemias. These probes can:

1. Be chromosome-specific that hybridize to satellite DNA sequences present at the centromere. These are especially applicable to cases with numerical abnormalities.
2. Hybridize to multiple sequences from a single chromosome: chromosome painting. These are particularly suitable for structural rearrangements (translocation). Examples include Philadelphia chromosome

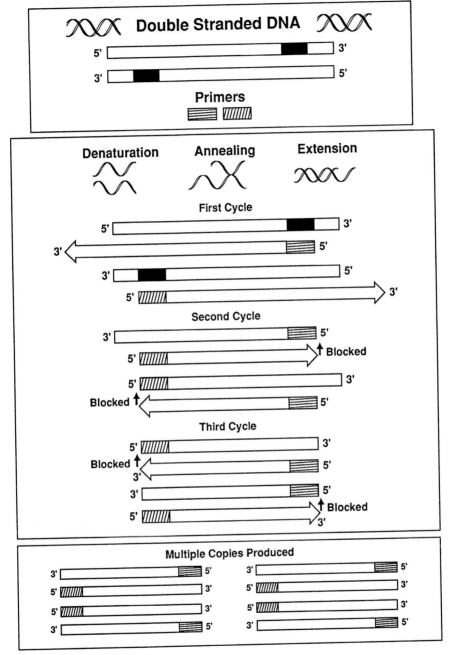

Figure 5.1. Polymerase chain reaction (PCR): amplification of DNA sequences.

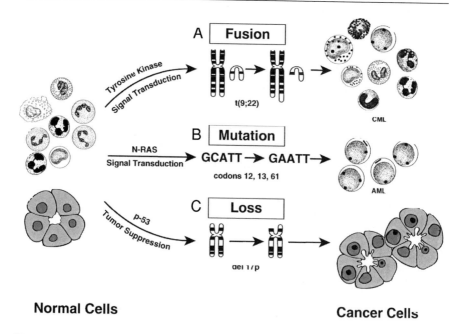

Normal Cells   **Cancer Cells**

Figure 5.2. Mechanisms of oncogenesis showing normal proto-oncogenes that are altered by (A) fusion, (B) mutation, and (C) loss. A. Depicts t(9;22) translocation (c-abl to bcr) in chronic myelogenous leukemia (CML). B. Shows a mutation in the N-RAS gene in acute myelogenous leukemia. C. Shows loss of the p-53 tumor suppressor gene in colon cancer. Tumor suppressor genes may also be disrupted by rearrangements and mutations. Usually more than one event is necessary to produce cancer. Left arrows indicate type of gene involved (top) and function of the gene product (bottom).

translocation t(9;22) of CML, the t(8;14), t(2;8), and t(8;22) seen in Burkitt's and 11q23 seen in ALL.

3. Be specific to a unique sequence.

In B-cell ALL, FISH detects translocation and numerical chromosomal abnormalities. Since hyperdiploid karyotype (greater than 50) is the most common cytogenetic abnormality in childhood ALL, centromere-specific probes (for chromosomes 1, 6, 8, 12, 17, 18, X and Y) detect numerical abnormalities. Although this finding carries a beneficial prognostic value, it is not associated with a specific phenotype. In AML, numerical chromosomal abnormalities occur with some frequency. The finding of a trisomy, as is in the case of trisomy 8, allows the documentation of clonal response to therapy. In addition, as in trisomy 8, FISH allows discrimination between a reactive and a neoplastic myeloid process in cases with questionable diagnosis. Similarly, the availability of centromeric and regional probe sets for chromosome 5 and 7 detect −7/del(7q) and 5q− assist in determining the presence of myelodysplastic syndrome (MDS) and therapy-related MDS, and evaluate these patients for minimal residual disease (MRD).

Table 5.1
Summary of Molecular Genetic Abnormalities

Diagnosis FAB Subtype	Molecular Genetics	Comment	Reference
Acute undifferentiated leukemia (AUL)	MPEX mRNA by RT-PCR bcr/abl fusion RT-PCR c-kit (CD117) product on myeloid precursors	Fewer AULs as technology advances	Leuk Res 1995;19:389–396 Leukemia 1995;9:1264–1275 Leukemia 1991;5:854–860
Hypoplastic/ aplastic ALL	No molecular genetic data available	PCR combined with high resolution denaturant gel electrophoretic analysis would be of value	Blood 1996;87:2506–2512 Cancer 1993;71:264–268
Granular ALL	TCR-γ and IgH rearrangement reported; PCR negative for *BCR-ABL* translocation	Additional cases need to be evaluated at molecular level.	Ann Hematol 1993;67:301–303
ALL with eosinophilia	t(5;14)(q31;q32) results in IgH gene and IL3 gene fusion and increased IL3 production	Eosinophils lack cytogenetic abnormality; stimulated by IL3	Blood 1990;76:285–289 J Clin Oncol 1987;5:382–390
ALL t (4;11)	t(4;11)(q21;q23) with rearrangement of ALL-1 gene on 11q23 and the AF-4 locus	Alteration of a very primitive homeobox gene at 11q23 with homology to sequences within Deosophilia trithorax genes	Cell 1992;71:701–708
ALL-hand mirror cell variant	Frequently germline in mixed leukemia hand mirror cell variants	Germline because cell in mixed leukemia hand mirror cell variant most likely a multipotential progenitor cell	Hematopathol Mol Hematol 1996;10:85–98 Am J Clin Pathol 1992;98:526–530
Aggressive NK cell leukemia	Germline for immunoglobulin and TCR genes. EBV associated leukemia	Germline as expected in aggressive NK cell leukemia which correlates with absence of TCR gene and IgH gene rearrangement in normal NK cells	Human Pathol 1994;25:953–960
AML-M0	Promiscuous IgH and TCR rearrangements. MPEX gene expression variable by in situ hybridization. C-kit expression not restricted to any FAB subtype	Findings in keeping with immature progenitor cell	Leukemia 1996;72:208–215 Diag Molecular Pathol 1995;4:212–219 Leukemia 1994;8:258–263

(Continued)

Table 5.1 *(Continued)*

Diagnosis FAB Subtype	Molecular Genetics	Comment	Reference
AML-M6 erythroleukemia	RT-PCR used to identify glycophorin A gene transcript in leukemic cell lines	Molecular studies not utilized much in erythroleukemia due to lack of specific chromosomal abnormality and heterogeneity of disorder	Vox Sang 1995;68:121–129
Acute basophilic leukemia	t(6;9)(p23;q34)DEK-CAN fusion produces p $165^{DEK-CAN}$ protein. t(6;9) can be diagnosed by Southern blot, and monitored by RNA-PCR	Translocation t(6;9) may also be present in AML M1, M4, MDS, and acute myelofibrosis. Some cases of ABL lack t(6;9). Not always associated with basophilia	Baillieres Clin Haematol 1992;5:857–879 Cancer Genet Cytogenet 1989;42:209–219
Eosinophilic leukemia/ hypereosinophilic syndrome	Possible gene regulating eosinophilia at 12p13 which is in proximity to oncogene c-Ki RAS 2	EL heterogeneous disorder as manifested by myriad of chromosomal abnormalities. HES should be non-clonal without cytogenetic abnormalities	Br J Haematol 1987;67:25–31 Blood 1985;66:1233–1240
Hypocellular AML	Molecular data sparse 5q-, monosomy 7, trisomy 8 seen. t(1;22) seen in children with hypocellular FAB AML M7	Future use of molecular genetic technique will be observed in these disorders	Blood 1992;79: 3325–3330 Exp Hematol 1987;15: 1134–1139 Blood 1991;77: 1397–1398
CD7+AML	Usually germline configuration by Southern blot with multidrug resistance phenotype	Clinical, karyotypic discrepancies. Southern blot analysis and MDR phenotype concordant in most studies	Am J Clin Pathol 1996;106:185–191 Cancer Genet Cytogenet 1994;73:69–74
AML inv 3(q21;q26)	EVI-1 gene and TPO gene map to 3q26. EVI-1 mRNA transcripts increased. TPO transcripts not increased	TPO gene transcription not activated and not responsible for the observed thrombocytosis in these cases	Br J Haematol 1995;91:425–427
Myeloid/NK acute leukemia	Lack promyelocytic/ RARα fusion transcript by RT-PCR. Lack TCR rearrangement. RT-PCR confirmed CD56 (neural cell adhesion molecule) in leukemic blasts	Important new entity with morphological features of FAB AML M3–M3v, but lacks t(15;17) and PML/RARα fusion gene. Does not respond to ATRA	Blood 1994;84:244–255
Bilineage/biphenotypic acute leukemia	MLL gene at 11q23 most common structural abnormality	Multipotent stem cell involved with early maturation arrest. Rearrangement of lymphocyte functional genes not used in lineage assignment because of overlay with AML	Ann Hematol 1991;62:16–21 Leukemia 1992;6(Suppl 2):1–6 Leukemia 1996;10:774–780

Probe sets for chromosomes 15 and 17 identify the characteristic translocation t(15,17) of acute promyelocytic leukemia (APL) FAB M3. Although the diagnosis of APL can be made by morphology, in some cases a rapid confirmation of the diagnosis may be indispensable to definitively establish the diagnosis before starting the patient on a specific therapeutic regimen. In addition, FISH can detect inversion of chromosome 16 in AML FAB M4 Eo variant. Figure 5.3 depicts how chromosomal aberrations can be detected in interphase nuclei by FISH.

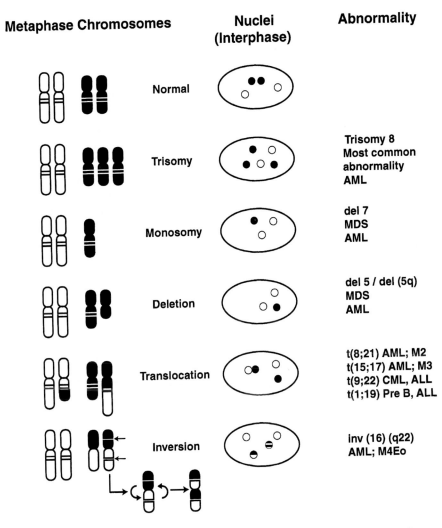

Figure 5.3. Schematic representations show how genomic features on metaphase chromosomes can detect interphase nuclei by fluorescent in situ hybridization (FISH). The metaphase chromosomes and their corresponding interphase nuclei are shown using chromosome specific probes. The signals detected by FISH are shown in the nuclei as circles.

Besides having probes specifically directed to alpha satellite DNA of a specific chromosome, each chromosome has unique repetitive sequences that enable one to label the entire chromosome. This whole chromosome paint probe allows the hematologist/hematopathologist to identify numerical abnormalities in chromosomes as well as translocations.

ACUTE UNDIFFERENTIATED LEUKEMIA (AUL)

With the impact of new technology, including detailed immunophenotyping, ultrastructural analysis, and RT-PCR, the number of AULs has declined considerably in the current literature.

Crisan and Anstett have developed a procedure for myeloperoxidase (MPEX) messenger ribonucleic acid (mRNA) detection by RT-PCR on routine hematology smears. They utilized the procedure in a retrospective analysis to evaluate the lineage of leukemic blasts in seven cases with morphology and cytochemistry consistent with AUL. Intriguingly, MPEX mRNA was detected in six cases, establishing the myeloid lineage of the blasts and the diagnosis of FAB AML M0. In the remaining case, the blasts were MPEX mRNA negative, supporting the initial diagnosis of AUL.

Besides MPEX mRNA detection to more clearly define AULs, Hattori et al. have used RT-mRNA to more clearly define the molecular genetics of an AUL. They described a patient with bcr/abl positive AUL derived from an acquired sideroblastic anemia secondary to ifosfamide treatment given for a preceding non-Hodgkin lymphoma of the lung. Although the Ph^1 was not detected through the patient's entire course, multiple chromosome abnormalities including 5q- and monosomy 7 were found at the stage of sideroblastic anemia. The RT-PCR analysis showed no bcr/abl fusion transcript at the time of diagnosis of the malignant lymphoma; however, the mRNA encoding the major bcr/abl fusion protein appeared in the stage of sideroblastic anemia. Finally, the mRNA encoding both major and minor bcr/abl was detected in the stage of AUL transformation. *MLL* (myeloid-lymphoid or mixed lineage leukemia) gene rearrangement was not discovered by RT-PCR analysis at any stage of the disease process. The authors concluded that the results may be direct evidence for the induction of the bcr/abl fusion gene by treatment with an alkylating agent (ifosfamide). Also, this case should alert the hematologic community to the possible potential of this drug to induce AUL.

Finally, Buhring et al. have reported that the product of the proto-oncogene c-Kit (p145/{C-KIT}) is a human bone marrow transmembrane protein receptor (CD117) of hemopoietic precursor cells that is expressed on a subset of acute nonlymphoblastic leukemic cells and not ALL cells. Although Wells et al. noted that CD117 was borne on most leukemic blasts of myeloid origin (87% AML, 80% myeloproliferative myeloid blast crisis, 75% of MDS) they also observed this marker in one of five cases of ALL. Therefore, this marker could not be used with certainty to clarify lineage in AUL.

ACUTE LYMPHOBLASTIC LEUKEMIA (ALL)

Hypocellular/Aplastic Acute Leukemia

Hypocellular/aplastic ALL is a rare condition that usually affects children. The ALL generally follows the recovery of normal blood counts and most commonly occurs within 6 months of the onset of aplastic anemia. Analysis of 23 case reports of hypocellular/aplastic ALL revealed several common characteristics including female sex, young age, and prevalence of fever, often associated with an infectious illness. Rare cases of hypoplastic anemia have developed in ALL secondary to human parvovirus (B19). Detailed cytogenetic analysis and molecular genetic studies of hypocellular/aplastic ALL have been nonexistent. Since more than 95% of precursor-B-ALL have IgH gene rearrangements and 85 to 90% of T-ALL have TCR-β or TCR-δ, molecular diagnostic techniques could be utilized to determine if leukemic clones are present in the hypoplastic/aplastic phase of the disease process. Southern blot analysis and conventional cytogenetic analysis would most likely be limited by sample size, but PCR, combined with high resolution denaturant gel electrophoretic analysis, could be utilized to establish clonality of rearranged VDJC bands. Careful analysis of such cases could give valuable new insights into the pathogenesis of hypocellular/aplastic ALL.

Granular ALL

Granular ALLs have shown no consistent cytogenetic associations, but several cases have been observed in children with Down syndrome and a number of others have been associated with the Philadelphia chromosome t(9;22)(q34;q11). Both findings would allow for special cytogenetic studies, i.e., FISH and molecular genetic analysis. Schwarzinger et al. evaluated an adult granular ALL with FAB L2 morphology and common-ALL immunologic phenotype by means of molecular genetic analysis. Cytogenetic analysis revealed a 46XY karyotype; however, molecular genetic investigation revealed TCR-δ and immunoglobulin heavy chain (IgH) rearrangements. No rearrangement was found at the TCR-β gene locus. Since some cases have been associated with the Ph[1], the authors performed PCR for the *BCR-ABL* translocation, which was negative. The patient's clinical course was uncomplicated and he achieved a complete remission within 4 weeks. Review of the literature on granular ALL revealed a lack of well-documented molecular genetic data as supplied by this case report.

ALL with Eosinophilia

Eosinophil proliferation is associated with B-lineage ALL with the t(5;14)(q31;q32). Meeker et al. reported on two cases of ALL with eosinophilia with the above karyotype that had been cloned from two leukemic samples. In both cases, this translocation joined the IgH gene and the interleukin-3 (IL3) gene. In one patient, excess IL3 mRNA was produced by the leukemic cells. In the other, serum IL3 levels were measured and shown to correlate with disease activity. There was no evidence of excess granulocyte-macrophage colony-stimulating factor (GM-CSF) or IL5 expression. The authors postulate that this subtype of leukemia may arise in part because of a chromosome translocation that activates the IL3 gene, resulting in autocrine and paracrine growth effects. Eosinophilia in these cases is thought to be reactive because the eosinophils lack the cytogenetic abnormalities.

Evidently, not all cases of ALL with eosinophilia manifest the t(5;14) chromosome rearrangement. The eosinophilia in these cases may be mild to marked, confused with a myeloproliferative disorder, and some patients demonstrate clinical manifestations of the hypereosinophilic syndrome. The eosinophilia generally resolves if a complete remission is accomplished, but may return with, or just prior to, relapse of the ALL. Eosinophilia has been reported in both FAB ALL L1 and L2.

ALL t(4;11)

The t(4;11)(q21;q23) is a nonrandom chromosomal abnormality that has been associated with FAB ALL L1 to L2, FAB AML M5a, and bilineage biphenotypic leukemia. Analysis of 107 infants less than 1 year of age with previously untreated ALL with 39 acceptable cytogenetic analyses revealed that 12 patients (31%) had a t(4;11)(q21;q23). These patients had a significantly shorter event-free survival than did the other patients with adequate cytogenetic analyses.

There has been a great interest concerning t(4;11)(q21;q23) because of the demonstration of the involvement of the *ALL*-1 (MLL) *gene* on band 11q23 of the *AF*-4 locus. This gene is rearranged in acute leukemias with interstitial deletions or reciprocal translocations between this region and chromosomes 1, 4, 6, 9, 10, or 19 (Fig. 5.4). The gene spans approximately 100Kb of DNA and contains at least 21 exons. It encodes a protein of more than 3910 amino acids containing three regions with homology to sequences within the Drosophila trithorax gene, including cysteine-rich regions that can be folded into six zinc fingerlike domains. The breakpoint cluster region within ALL-1 (MLL) gene spans 8 Kb and encompasses several small exons, most of which begin in the same phase of the open reading frame. The t(4;11) results in two reciprocal fusion products coding for chimeric proteins derived from ALL-1 (MLL) and from a gene on chromosome 4. This suggests that each 11q23 abnormality gives rise to a specific oncogenic fusion protein. Furthermore, the presence of heptameric and nonameric sequences close to the breakpoints suggests that a mistake of the recombinase system physiologically active in pre-B elements may be responsible for the translocation. The involvement of the band 11q23 in a group of leukemias secondary to the use of topoisomerase II inhibitors (antracyclines, mitox-

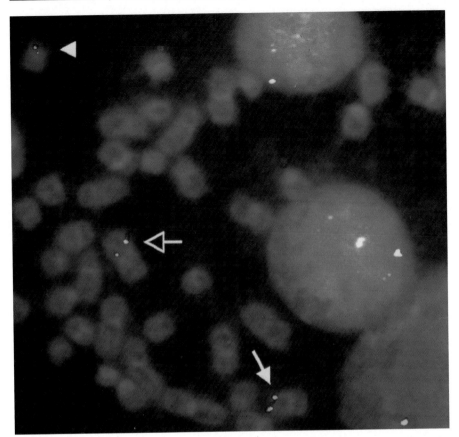

Figure 5.4. A. Metaphase demonstrating FISH with the MLL probe labeled with FITC on cells with ins(10;11)(p12;q13q23). The intact chromosome 11 (solid arrow) shows normal hybridization signal intensity, while the derived 10 demonstrates a signal of decreased size (open arrow). The derivative 11 also demonstrates a reduced signal, indicating that the MLL gene was disrupted by the translocation (arrowhead). Patient had RAEB-IT. Courtesy of Ruth Blough. B. Whole chromosome 11 paint analysis of a metaphase spread from the previous patient, confirming insertion of chromosome 11 material into the short arm of chromosome 10 (open arrow). The normal chromosome 11 is indicated by the solid arrow. The paint probe is labeled with FITC. Courtesy of Ruth Blough, Linda Shepard.

antrone, or epipodophylotoxin derivatives VP16 or VM26) and cyclophosphamide suggests that this region of genome could be particularly susceptible to chemical agents. These agents have also been implicated in the pathogenesis of secondary AML with 11q23 rearrangements.

PCR has been used in ALL with t(4;11) to detect MRD. The results of PCR in evaluation of MRD has varied with different leukemias. Therefore, the clinical relevance of MRD detection should be evaluated separately for each type of leukemia as significant prognostic differences between disease entities exist.

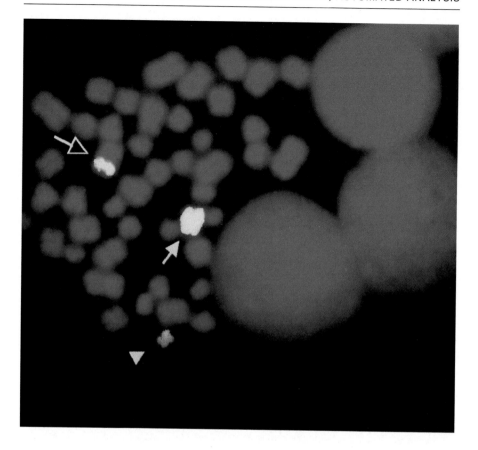

ALL-Hand Mirror Variant (HMV)

Molecular analysis of cases of ALL-HMV are sparse in the literature. Mazur et al. reported on 14 adults with ALL-HMV that appeared to be a distinctive clinicopathologic entity. The group showed a female predominance, a relatively indolent early clinical course, and a failure to achieve a complete remission with chemotherapy. Phenotypically, the hand mirror cells (HMCs) were null cells, Ia positive, TdT positive, and stained positive for acid phosphatase. Although gene rearrangement analysis was not performed on these early cases, the authors alluded to the fact that their cases were most likely committed to B-cell differentiation at the gene level. Unfortunately, none of these cases were studied with today's modern technology.

More recently, Kovarik et al. investigated a case of ALL-HMV by means of modern technology and demonstrated the blast cells to be pre B cells (CD19+ and TdT+) that also expressed myeloid antigens CD13 and CD33. Cytogenetic studies revealed a t(11;19) translocation previously described in biphenotypic leukemias. Molecular genetic analysis revealed a clonal rearrangement of the IgH gene that comprised approximately 5% of the cells assayed. No detectable rearrangements or deletions of the T-cell receptor-beta gene or Ig kappa light chain gene were noted. The authors stressed the importance of investigating leukemic cases with HMCs for possible mixed lineage.

More recently, Zucker et al. reported another case of acute biphenotypic leukemia with mixed blast morphology and combined myeloid and T-lymphoid features. Surprisingly, the small leukemia blasts demonstrated hand mirror configuration, but the larger blasts with granules and Auer rods failed to reveal such morphology. Cytogenetic analysis of the bone marrow revealed a complex translocation involving chromosomes 13, 20, and 22. Gene rearrangement analysis revealed no clonal rearrangements of TCR-β, TCR-γ or IgH genes.

Most recently, Wibowo et al. reported two additional patients with numerous HMCs in the bone marrow. Both demonstrated a mixed immunophenotype with expression of myeloid and T-lymphoid features. Interestingly, both strongly expressed CD2 (adhesion molecule) and CD7. Review of the literature uncovered additional cases of acute mixed leukemias-HMV with strong expression of CD2, CD7, and CD11b, suggesting a unique subset. Genotypic analysis of the two cases revealed germline configuration for kappa light chain, IgH, and TCR in case 1 and rearranged bands with TCR-β and germline configuration for kappa light chain and IgH in case 2.

Even though HMC leukemias represent a heterogeneous group of disorders, thorough investigation of each case is indicated to correctly place them into appropriate subsets. Such classification will help in diagnosis, prognosis, and treatment.

Aggressive NK Cell Leukemia (ANKCL)

Three distinct clinical syndromes occur in patients with increased numbers of circulating large granular lymphocytes (LGL). Patients with T-LGL leukemia have clonal proliferations of CD3+LGL, typically associated with chronic neutropenia and autoimmune features. Aggressive NK-LGL is characterized by clonal CD3-LGL proliferation with an acute clinical presentation marked by massive hepatosplenomegaly and systemic illness. Most patients with increased numbers of CD3-LGL, however, do not have clinical features of aggressive NK-LGL leukemia, but have a chronic clinical course.

The Epstein-Barr virus (EBV) has been implicated in the aggressive NK-LGL leukemia. Gelb et al. described the first case of EBV-associated aggressive NK-LGL leukemia in the United States in a 29-year-old woman of Japanese descent. She developed EBV infection after a blood transfusion as indicated by a rise in antibody titers. Peripheral blood and bone marrow aspirate smears demonstrated increased LGLs. The clinical course was rapid and death followed colonic rupture. Necropsy findings included bone marrow lymphocytosis and erythrophagocytosis, a mononucleosis-like lymphadenitis, atypical hepatitis with a mixed predominately T-cell infiltrate, interstitial pneumonitis, and multiorgan system vasculitis with perforation of the transverse colon. EBV transcripts were identified in lymphocytes infiltrating liver and peripheral nerve by in situ hybridization. In addition, Southern blot analyses showed monoclonal bands superimposed on oligoclonal ladders of EBV termini in the liver and lymph nodes. The identical episomal form of EBV was found in the bone marrow, lymph nodes, and liver. No immunoglobulin, TCR-β, or TCR-γ gene rearrangements were identified. This is as would be expected since NK-LGLs have all TCR and IgH genes in germline configuration, which correlates with the absence of TCR gene and IgH gene rearrangement in normal NK cells.

Recently, Brody et al. have reported an acute agranular CD4+ NK cell leukemia with a unique phenotype (CD3−, CD56+, CD4+, CD15+) in which, unlike other aggressive NK cell leukemias, EBV was negative. Also, there was no evidence of human herpes virus 6. The viruses were studied by means of Southern blot analysis, PCR, and in vitro culturing with inducing agents. Immunoglobulin and T-cell receptor genes were germline as expected. Such findings suggest that different etiologic mechanisms are operating in the agranular NK cell leukemias.

ACUTE MYELOID LEUKEMIA (AML)

AML M0

FAB AML M0 frequently bears "stem cell" markers such as CD34, HLA-DR, TdT, and CD7. Molecular analysis reveals frequent immunoglobulin and TCR rearrangements. Also, FAB AML M0 very frequently carries cytogenetic abnormalities common to MDS or secondary AML, such as −5/5q− or −7/7q− deletions or complex karyotypes. Also, FAB AML M0 is frequently associated with the multidrug resistance (MDR) phenotype. MDR has been found to be linked to stem cell features, especially in MDS.

Since the M0 cells are considered immature hematopoietic progenitors, studies utilizing CD117 have been undertaken by a number of investigators. CD117 is a transmembrane protein receptor encoded by the c-kit proto-oncogene. The CD117 ligand is stem cell factor, an important hematopoietic regulator. CD117 is present on approximately 4% of normal bone marrow mononuclear cells and in acute myelogenous leukemia and chronic myelogenous leukemia in myeloid blast crisis, but rarely in ALL. Reuss-Borst et al. studied 95 acute leukemias with the monoclonal antibody 17F11 directed against the c-kit structure. They found 41/47 AML and 6/8 CML blast crisis that were positive for c-kit expression; whereas all 40 ALLs were negative. C-kit was not restricted to any particular, undifferentiated subtype, but found in 9/9 AML M0/M1, 18/19 AML M2, 0/1 AML M3, 11/13 AML M4, and 3/5 AML M5 subtypes. Wells et al. investigated 45 cases of acute leukemia to determine if immature progenitor markers CD117 and CD34 correlate. Interestingly, no correlation was demonstrated in this study. Recent studies have mapped the c-kit oncogene to chromosome 4, an association that should be further investigated.

Traweek et al. have investigated the association of MPEX and myeloid antigen expression in AML; particularly at the early stages of myeloid differentiation. They used in situ hybridization to evaluate MPEX expression in myeloid leukemia cell lines and a variety of well-characterized acute leukemias. Strong positivity for MPEX mRNA was detected in the myeloid cell line HL-60 and in 22 of 27 AMLs (3 AML M0, 4 AML M1, 8 AML M2, 5 AML M4, and 2 AML M5a). No MPEX gene expression was detected in 3 AML M0, 1 AML 5a, 1 AML M7, and 5 ALLs. Ultrastructural studies for MPEX activity were performed on 4 AML M0; one leukemia showed both gene expression and cytochemical activity, whereas two others contained neither MPEX transcripts nor enzyme. Weak MPEX gene expression was evident in 1 AML M0 that was negative for enzymatic activity by electron microscopy. The authors state that MPEX gene expression can be detected by in situ hybridization in about half of AML M0, supporting their presumed myelocytic derivation.

AML M6-Erythroleukemia

Molecular genetic diagnostic techniques have not been utilized in erythroleukemia. This relates to the fact that the disorder is heterogeneous and no specific chromosomal abnormality has been described. Also, the diagnosis is usually established by morphology, cytochemistry, immunohistochemistry, and flow cytometric analysis. The latter study identifies glycophorin A, a specific marker for red cell precursors. In our hands, glycophorin A has not been helpful in flow cytometric analysis due to the immaturity of the red cell precursors found in erythroleukemia.

Du Pont et al. used purified cDNAs and RNAs isolated from peripheral blood and erythroleukemia cell lines, HEL, and K562 to develop an RT-PCR technique for amplifying the glycophorin A gene transcripts. The authors stated that the method permitted sensitive identification of glycophorin A gene transcripts in these cells and confirms glycophorin A protein expression in the erythroleukemia cell lines. RT-PCR amplification of glycophorin A gene transcripts may have diagnostic and prognostic implications in erythroleukemia in the future.

Of interest, are the findings of Wang et al. who performed RT-PCR to evaluate the chimeric transcript *AML1/MTG8* that resulted from a t(8;21) reciprocal chromosomal translocation. They studied 41 patients with FAB AML M2b. Thirty-seven patients with the t(8;21) demonstrated the chimeric transcript. In the remaining four patients with a normal karyotype, *AML1/MTG*8 fusion mRNA and/or rearrangements of *AML*1 and *MTG*8 genes were detected. Evaluation of 31 patients with other types of AML revealed the abnormality in only one patient with FAB AML M6. The authors offered no explanation as to why such a genetic abnormality uniquely associated with FAB M2b should be found in erythroleukemia.

Acute Basophilic Leukemia (ABL)

The leukemias that involve the basophilic lineage are heterogeneous in their molecular genetics, rare, and not well characterized. One subset of FAB AML M2 baso demonstrates an increase in the number of basophils, granulocytic maturation, and variable blastic infiltrates with basophilic granules. This basophilic leukemia is associated with t(6;9)(p23;q34); however, this translocation has also been reported in patients with acute myelofibrosis, MDS, and AML with and without increased marrow basophils. For these reasons, Cuneo et al. have suggested that the t(6;9) is associated with a multipotent stem cell. The t(6;9) that characterizes the FAB AML M2 baso fuses the 3' part of a gene located on chromosome 9q34, *CAN*, to the 5' part of a gene located on chromosome 6p23, *DEK*. On the 6p− chromosome, the resulting *DEK-CAN* fusion gene is transcribed into a leukemic-specific 5.5 Kb chimeric mRNA that encodes a fusion protein (p165$^{DEK-CAN}$ protein) that is involved in the control of DNA transcription. No transcription could be detected from the reciprocal *CAN-DEK* fusion on chromosome 9q+. Von Lindern et al. analyzed 17 t(6;9) AML cases and showed that the translocation breakpoints occur in a single intron of 7.5 Kb in the *CAN* gene (ICB9) and in a single intron of 9Kb in the *DEK* gene (ICB6). As a result, the presence of a t(6;9) in blood or bone marrow may be determined by Southern blot analysis. Moreover, the result of the translocation is an invariable *DEK-CAN* transcript that can be sensitively monitored by RNA-PCR. Surprisingly, a *SET-CAN* fusion gene has been found in leukemic cells from a patient with AUL. Like *CAN*, *SET* is located on chromosome 9q34, which explains the apparently normal karyotype of the leukemic cells.

Basophilia in AML has also been associated with abnormalities of the short arm of chromosome 12. In addition, basophils may be increased in the blast crisis of CML. Peterson et al. have described eight cases of ABL identified on the basis of ultrastructural analysis. Cytogenetic studies showed the cases to be heterogeneous; three had a Ph[1], none had t(6;9). Such reports emphasize the heterogeneous nature of ABL and demonstrate the future need for more molecular genetic studies.

Eosinophilic Leukemia (EL)/Hypereosinophilic Syndromes (HES)

Molecular genetic studies have been rather limited in EL. This relates to the fact that a little more than 100 cases have been reported in the literature and confusion exists concerning diagnostic criteria that remains elusive because some cases with large numbers of immature cells and the putative eosinophilic blasts have not been fully characterized. Also, eosinophilia may be observed in three broad categories: 1) cases associated with non-neoplastic conditions; 2) idiopathic cases, where eosinophilia may be protracted and unexplained (hyper-eosinophilic syndrome); and 3) heterogeneous group, where eosinophilia either precedes, succeeds, or is part of a malignant process. EL belongs to this last group and proof of a clonal cytogenetic abnormality is now considered confirmatory evidence of leukemia. Although a variety of chromosomal abnormalities, including the Ph[1], trisomy 7, 8, 9, and 10, 9q−, translocation abnormalities of 12p13, t(10;11), t(5;11), t(8;21), a short Y chromosome, and isochromosome 17 have been observed and catalogued by Keene et al.; no specific marker appears to be present. Therefore, studies involving Southern blot, PCR, and FISH would need to be individualized to each case. Despite this great cytogenetic variation in EL, Saito et al. established a cell line from a case of EL that demonstrated surface Ia antigen, the myeloid antigens IF10 and CD33, and membrane receptors for IL2, and the Tac antigen. This conundrum of information prompted the belief that EL does in fact exist as a distinct entity. Keene et al. have demonstrated translocation abnormalities of chromosome 12p13 in cases of acute EL, Ph[1] negative myeloproliferative disease, and ALL. They speculate that a gene regulating eosinophil production may be located at this site, which is in proximity to the oncogene c-Ki RAS 2. The only well-documented case of acute secondary EL is reported by Maeda et al., and developed 8 years after melphalan treatment for multiple myeloma in a 71-year-old woman. The cytogenetic abnormalities included a 5q− and a monosomy 7, being similar to those observed in other patients with chemotherapy-induced secondary AML.

Hypocellular AML

Molecular genetic studies of patients with hypocellular AML are, for the most part, nonexistent. The studies of Appelbaum et al. and Moormeier et al. concerning cytogenetics in separating hypocellular MDS from acquired aplastic anemia was discussed in Chapter 4; however, the chromosomal abnormalities frequently seen in MDS and AML including deletion of the long arm of chromosome 5, monosomy 7, and trisomy 8 were seen in 7(4%) of 183 patients initially diagnosed as aplastic anemia. Molecular probes employing FISH analysis could be used to an advantage in such cases. Lion et al. have reported the occurrence of a t(1;22) in children with hypocellular AML. The translocation occurred in 5 of 445 (1.1%) of children with newly diagnosed AML. The t(1;22) was restricted to FAB AML M7. Of interest was the finding that the translocation occurred in 5/18 (27.8%) of children and 4/6 (66.7%) of infants with FAB AML M7. This translocation will require future studies to enable investigators to apply molecular genetic techniques to diagnostic and prognostic advantages.

CD7 positive AML

CD7 is expressed in 10 to 30% of AML cases, more frequently in FAB AML M0, M1, and M5a. There is much controversy in the literature concerning prognostic significance, clinical characteristics, and even cytogenetic findings.

Launder et al. evaluated 74 cases of AML for lymphoid antigen expression and gene rearrangement. Sixteen of the 74 cases (22%) were identified as lymphoid antigen+ AML. Of these, the T cell associated markers CD7, CD2, and CD5 were expressed on 7(44%), 6(38%), and 4(25%), respectively. B cell associated markers CD19 and CD20 were expressed on two cases (13%) and one case (6%), respectively. Southern blot analysis revealed that the majority of these cases revealed no Ig or TCR gene rearrangement. The authors concluded that expression of CD7, CD2, CD5 in otherwise straightforward AML should not be taken as evidence of lymphoid lineage commitment and does not warrant a diagnosis of acute mixed leukemia. In support of these findings, Shimamoto et al. studied six patients with CD7+ AML. All but one had germline configuration of the TCR genes and IgH genes; however, all did not have detectable recombinase activating gene-1 activity by RT-PCR. Contrary to a recent report by Del Poeta et al. who reported abnormal complex karyotypes, cytogenetic analysis revealed normal karyotypes in all the cases.

Yamaguchi et al. investigated 104 cases of AML and 30 with ALL for P-glycoprotein/MDR1 by means of a Rhodamine 123 efflux test and made estimations with data obtained by RT-PCR method. In AML, frequent p-glycoprotein/MDR1 expression was associated with the expression of CD7 or c-kit (CD117), which was characteristic of a hematopoietic stem cell.

The discrepancies in the prognostic significance, clinical characteristics and cytogenetic findings in numerous studies supports a stem cell disorder that is behaving in a variety of different ways. Contrary to this discordance are the uniform findings that most cases have malignant cells that are in germline configuration and demonstrate an MDR phenotype.

AML inv 3(q21;q26)

There has been an association between AML or MDS presenting with normal platelet counts or thrombocytosis, striking dysmegakaryopoiesis abnormalities of the long arm of chromosome 3, and an unfavorable prognosis. These cases may have platelet counts in excess of 1000×10^9/L. Furthermore, they are difficult to classify and have demonstrated variable FAB classification: AML M1, AML M4, AML M6.

Bouscary et al. have studied four patients with typical 3q21;q26 at the molecular level. Karyotypic analysis revealed inv (3)(q21;q26) in three cases and t(3;3)(q21;q26) in one case. Leukemic cells from these cases ectopically express the *EVI*-1 gene that maps to human chromosome 3q26;q27. Also, the thrombopoietin (TPO) gene maps to human chromosome 3q26. Recently, TPO has been cloned and shown to be the major hormone stimulating both megakaryopoiesis and thrombopoiesis. Interestingly, Bouscary et al. found high levels of EVI-1 transcripts detected in mRNA isolated from the bone marrow cells of these patients by Northern blot analysis; however, no TPO transcripts were detectable by RT-PCR on the same mRNA samples. The authors concluded that TPO transcription is not activated in patients with 3q26 chromosomal abnormality, and that abnormal TPO production is not responsible for the observed thrombocytosis.

Myeloid/NK-Leukemia

There is a form of myeloid/natural killer cell acute leukemia that has been potentially misdiagnosed as FAB AML M3. In an analysis of 350 cases of adult de novo AML, Scott et al. identified 20 cases (6%) with a unique immunophenotype: CD33+, CD56+, CD11a+, CD13 lo, CD15 lo, CD34+lo−, HLA-DR−, and CD16−. Multicolor flow cytometric assays confirmed the coexpression of myeloid (CD33, CD13, CD15) and NK cell associated (CD56) antigens in each case; whereas, RT-PCR assays confirmed the identity of CD56 (neural cell adhesion molecule). None of the cases showed clonal rearrangement of genes encoding the T-cell receptor (TCR beta, gamma, delta). Of diagnostic importance was the finding that the leukemic blasts were remarkably similar to those of APL (FAB AML M3); particularly the microgranular variant (FAB AML M3v). Nevertheless, all 20 cases lacked the t(15;17) and 17 cases tested lacked the promyelocytic/retinoic acid receptor alpha (RAR alpha) fusion transcript in RT-PCR assays; 12 cases had 46, XX or 46, XY karyotypes, whereas two cases had abnormalities of chromosome 17q: 1 with del(17) q25 and the other with t(11;17) (q23;q21) and the promyelocytic leukemia zinc finger/RAR alpha fusion transcript. All cases tested (6/20), including the case with t(11;17), failed to differentiate in vitro in response to all-trans retinoic acid (ATRA) suggesting that these cases may account for some so called APLs that have not shown a clinical response to ATRA. Correct identification of such cases is most important since they do not respond to ATRA.

BILINEAGE/BIPHENOTYPIC ACUTE LEUKEMIA

Most schemes to establish a diagnosis of bilineage or biphenotypic leukemia heavily utilize immunophenotyping. Although, in 1991, Catovsky et al. proposed a scoring system that depended mostly on immunophenotypic findings for biphenotypic leukemia, they also included the results of IgH and TCR rearrangement analysis (see Chapter 3). This was quickly modified by elevating the minimum score for lineage to 2.5 and by excluding data on rearrangement of lymphocyte functional genes. The latter exclusion was related to the fact that the high incidence of IgH and TCR gene rearrangements was observed in AMLs with expression of lymphoid markers.

Yu et al. noted that rearrangement of the MLL gene frequently occurs in patients with monocytic, lymphoid, and biphenotypic leukemias. At the molecular level, these patients demonstrate an 11q23 breakpoint that fuses the MLL gene (also named *ALL-1*, *HRX*, *Htrx* 1) to a second partner gene. By means of RT-PCR and Southern blot analysis, they found that 7 of 34 patients with MLL gene rearrangement had a tandem partial duplication of exons 2 to 6 or 2 to 8 of the MLL gene with an unfavorable prognosis. Other investigators noted marked heterogeneity in the pattern of rearrangement of antigen receptor genes in mixed lineage leukemias. They observed that re-arrangements of the MLL gene were confined to the leukemias that demon-strated lineage infidelity. They concluded that mixed lineage and bipheno-typic leukemias accumulate pathogenetic lesions that are distinct from B and T cell ALL, and that ALL in developing countries includes molecular enti-ties similar to those in developed countries. Williams et al. noted that in the majority of acute leukemias, including those with myeloid phenotypes, re-vealed characteristics of early lymphoid differentiation. They demonstrated that expression of TdT mRNA and sterile transcription at both Ig and TCR loci (transcription without gene rearrangement) was unexpectedly common in both acute biphenotypic and myelogenous leukemia, and occurred in the absence of phenotypic lymphoid differentiation. Kovarik et al. noted heavy chain gene rearrangement in an adult acute mixed leukemia with a t(11;19) and numerous HMCs. They suggested that the finding of large numbers of HMCs in the bone marrow should warrant analysis for a mixed im-munophenotype. Finally, Ridge et al. described a case of neonatal mixed lin-eage leukemia that presented with a dominant B progenitor lymphoblast population plus a minor monocytic component. The two cell lines (bilineal) were monoclonal since both showed identical rearrangement in the MLL gene and a shared rearrangement of one IgH allele. Although cytogenetic studies have demonstrated that chromosome 11, region 11q23 is the most common structural abnormality, t(9;22)(q34,q11), trisomy 13, and aberra-tions of chromosome 44 at band q32 have been reported in these leukemias. Finally, cytogenetic and molecular genetic analysis strongly supports the view that bilineal/biphenotypic acute leukemia involve a multipotent stem cell and an early maturation arrest.

BIBLIOGRAPHY

Articles

Appelbaum FR, Borall J, Storb R, et al. Clonal cytogenetic abnormalities in patients with otherwise typical aplastic anemia. Exp Hematol 1987;15:1134–1139.
Bouscary D, Fontenay-Roupie M, Chretien S, et al. Thrombopoietin is not responsible for the thrombocytosis observed in patients with acute myeloid leukemias and the 3q21q26 syndrome. Br J Haematol 1995;91(2):425–427.
Brody JP, Allen S, Schulman P, et al. Acute agranular CD4-positive natural killer cell leukemia. Comprehensive clinicopathologic studies including virologic and in vitro culture with inducing agents. Cancer 1995;75(10):2474–2483.

Buhring HJ, Ullrich A, Schaudt K, et al. The product of the proto-oncogene c-kit (P145c-kit) is a human bone marrow surface antigen of hemopoietic precursor cells which is expressed on a subset of acute nonlymphoblastic leukemic cells. Leukemia 1991;5:854–860.

Catovsky D, Matutes E. The classification of acute leukemia. Leukemia 1992;6(Suppl 2):1–6.

Choi Y, Greenberg SJ, Du TL, et al. Clonal evolution in B-lineage acute lymphoblastic leukemia by contemporaneous VH-VH gene replacements and VH-DJH gene rearrangements. Blood 1996;87(6):2506–2512.

Crisan D, Anstett MJ. Myeloperoxidase mRNA detection for lineage determination of leukemic blasts: retrospective analysis. Leukemia 1995;9(7):1264–1275.

Cuneo A, Kerim S, Vandenberghe E, et al. Translocation t(6;9) occurring in acute myelofibrosis, myelodysplastic syndrome, and acute nonlymphocytic leukemia suggests multipotent stem cell involvement. Cancer Genet Cytogenet 1989;42(2):209–219.

Del Poeta G, Stasi R, Venditti A, et al. CD7 expression in acute myeloid leukemia. Leuk Lymphoma 1995;17:111–119.

DuPont BR, Grant SG, Oto SH, et al. Molecular characterization of glycophorin A transcripts in human erythroid cells using RT-PCR, allele-specific restriction, and sequencing. Vox Sang 1995;68(2):121–129.

Gelb AB, van de Rijn M, Regula DP Jr, et al. Epstein-Barr virus-associated natural killer-large granular lymphocyte leukemia. Hum Pathol 1994;25(9):953–960.

Grimaldi JC, Meker TC. The t(5;14) chromosomal translocation in a case of acute lymphocytic leukemia joins the interleukin-3 gene to the immunoglobulin heavy chain gene. Blood 1989;73(8):2081–2085.

Gu Y, Nakamura T, Alder H, et al. The t(4;11) chromosome translocation of human acute leukemias fuses the ALL-1 gene, related to Drosophila trithorax, to the AF-4 gene. Cell 1992;71(4):701–708.

Hamdy N, Bhatia K, Shaker H, et al. Molecular epidemiology of acute lymphoblastic leukemia in Egypt. Leukemia 1995;9(1):194–202.

Hattori M, Tanaka M, Yamazaki Y, et al. Detection of major and minor bcr/abl fusion gene transcripts in a patient with acute undifferentiated leukemia secondary to treatment with an alkylating agent. Leuk Res 1995;19(6):389–396.

Heerema NA, Arthur DC, Sather H, et al. Cytogenetic features of infants less than 12 months of age at diagnosis of acute lymphoblastic leukemia: impact of the 11q23 breakpoint on outcome: a report of the Children's Cancer Group. Blood 1994;83(8):2274–2284.

Keene P, Mendelow B, Pinto MR, et al. Abnormalities of chromosome 12p13 and malignant proliferation of eosinophils: a nonrandom association. Br J Haematol 1987;67(1):25–31.

Kovarik P, Shrit MA, Yuen B, et al. Hand mirror variant of adult acute lymphoblastic leukemia. Am J Clin Pathol 1992;98(5):526–530.

Launder TM, Bray RA, Stempora L, et al. Lymphoid-associated antigen expression by acute myeloid leukemia. Am J Clin Pathol 1996;106(2):185–191.

Lion T, Haas OA, Harbott J, et al. The translocation t(1;22) (p13;q13) is a nonrandom marker specifically associated with acute megakaryocytic leukemia in young children. Blood 1992;79(12):3325–3330.

Maeda K, VanSlyck EJ, VanDyke DL. Multiple myeloma terminating in acute eosinophilic leukemia. Cancer Genet Cytogenet 1985;16(1):81–89.

Mazur EM, Wittels EG, Schiffman FJ, et al. Hand mirror cell lymphoid leukemia in adults: a distinct clinicopathologic syndrome. Case report and literature review. Cancer 1986;57:92–99.

Meeker TC, Hardy D, Willman C, et al. Activation of the interleukin-3 gene by chromosome translocation in acute lymphocytic leukemia with eosinophilia. Blood 1990;76(2):285–289.

Moormeier JA, Rubin CM, LeBeau MM, et al. Trisomy 6: a recurring cytogenetic abnormality associated with marrow hypoplasia. Blood 1991;77:1397–1398.

Peterson LC, Parkin JL, Arthur DC, et al. Acute basophilic leukemia: a clinical morphologic and cytogenetic study of eight cases. Am J Clin Pathol 1991;96:160–170.

Reuss-Borst MA, Buhring HJ, Schmidt H, et al. AML: immunophenotypic heterogeneity and prognostic significance of c-kit expression. Leukemia 1994;8(2):258–263.

Ridge SA, Cabrera ME, Ford AM, et al. Rapid intraclonal switch of lineage dominance in congenital leukemia with a MLL gene rearrangement. Leukemia 1995;9(12):2023–2026.

Saito H, Bourinbaiar A, Ginsburg M, et al. Establishment and characterization of a new human eosinophilic leukemia cell line. Blood 1985;66:1233–1240.

Scott AA, Head DR, Kopecky KJ, et al. HLA-DR–, CD33+, CD56+, CD16– myeloid/natural killer cell acute leukemia: a previously unrecognized form of acute leukemia potentially misdiagnosed as French-American-British acute myeloid leukemia-M3. Blood 1994;84(1):244–255.

Traweek ST, Liu J, Braziel RM, et al. Detection of myeloperoxidase gene expression in minimally differentiated acute myelogenous leukemia (AML-M0) using in situ hybridization. Diagn Mol Pathol 1995;4(3):212–219.

Wang J, Xiao Z, Hao Y. Rearrangements and fusion gene of AML1 and MTG8 in acute myeloid leukemia M2b. Chung-Hua I Hsueh Tsa Chih (Chinese Medical Journal) 1995;75(7):399–402, 445.

Wells SJ, Bray RA, Stempora LL, et al. CD117/CD34 expression in leukemic blasts. Am J Clin Pathol 1996;106(2):192–195.

Williams L, Moscinski LC. Sterile transcription of immunoglobulin/T-cell receptor genes and other evidence of early lymphoid differentiation in acute myelogenous leukemia. Leukemia 1993;7(9):1423–1431.

Yamaguchi M, Mizutani M, Miwa H, et al. [P-glycoprotein expression in hematological malignancies.] Rinsho Ketsueki 1995;36(6):567–572.

Yu M, Honoki K, Andersen J, et al. MLL tandem duplication and multiple splicing in adult acute myeloid leukemia with normal karyotype. Leukemia 1996;10(5):774–780.

Zucker ML, Plapp FB, Rachel JM, et al. An adult case of acute biphenotypic leukemia with characteristic mixed morphology. Mo Med 1993;90:601–604.

Review Articles

Amadori S, Venditti A, Del Poeta G, et al. Minimally differentiated acute myeloid leukemia (AML-M0): a distinct clinicobiologic entity with poor prognosis. Ann Hematol 1996;72(4):208–215.

Auxenfants E, Morel P, Lai JL, et al. Secondary acute lymphoblastic leukemia with t(4;11): report on two cases and review of the literature. Ann Hematol 1992;65(3):143–146.

Catovsky D, Matutes E, Buccheri V, et al. A classification of acute leukemia for the 1990s. Ann Hematol 1991;62(1):16–21.

Drexler HG, Borkhardt A, Janssen JW. Detection of chromosomal translocations in leukemia-lymphoma cells by polymerase chain reaction. Leuk Lymphoma 1995;19(5-6):359–380.

Hogan TF, Koss W, Murgo AJ, et al. Acute lymphoblastic leukemia with chromosomal 5;14 translocation and hypereosinophilia: case report and literature review. J Clin Oncol 1987;5(3):382–390.

Keung YK, Kaplan B, Douer D. Biphenotypic M0 acute myeloid leukemia with trisomy-4. Leuk Lymphoma 1994;14(1-2):181–184.

Loughran TP Jr. Clonal diseases of large granular lymphocytes. Blood 1993;82(1):1–14.

Matloub YH, Brunning RD, Arthur DC, et al. Severe aplastic anemia preceding acute lymphoblastic leukemia. Cancer 1993;71(1):264–268.

Schwarzinger I, Fodinger M, Scherrer R, et al. Hypergranular acute lymphoblastic leukemia (ALL). Report of a case and review of the literature. Ann Hematol 1993;67(6):301–303.

Shimamoto T, Ohyashiki JH, Ohyashiki K, et al. Clinical and biologic characteristics of CD7+ acute myeloid leukemia. Our experience and literature review. Cancer Genet Cytogenet 1994;73(1):69–74.

von Lindern M, Fornerod M, Soekarman N, et al. Translocation t(6;9) in acute non-lymphocytic leukemia results in the formation of a DEK-CAN fusion gene. Baillieres Clin Haematol 1992;5(4):857–879.

Wibowo A, Pankowsky D, Mikhael A, et al. Adult acute leukemia: hand mirror cell variant. Hematopath Mol Hematol 1996;10:85–98.

CHAPTER 6

Cytokines

GENERAL COMMENTS

The mechanisms that control growth, differentiation, and division of hematopoietic cells are extremely complex and poorly understood. In the 1960s, culture techniques utilizing semisolid microenvironments were developed that successfully supported the clonal growth of normal hematopoietic progenitor cells. With the arrival of such systems, it was shown that specific glycoproteins are required for the survival, proliferation, and induction of lineage-specific differentiation in both normal and leukemic cells. Originally, these growth factors, cytokines, were obtained from cultured lymphocytes, requiring laborious purification; however, more recently, manufacturing through recombinant gene technology has expedited the clinical testing of these substances. These cell growth and development regulating factors have been employed either for their properties of tumor cell inhibition or their ability to stimulate normal hematopoiesis, and, thereby, reduce the toxicity of conventional cytotoxic therapies. The progress in this area has been so expeditious that new activities and factors are being added almost daily.

Initially, growth factors defined concerning the myeloid differentiation pathways were termed *colony-stimulating-factors* (*CSFs*) and those generally involving lymphoid pathways were designated *interleukins* (*ILs*). Nevertheless, as information accumulated, it became increasingly obvious that *CSFs*, *ILs*, and oncogenes were inextricably intertwined in cell growth, differentiation, and division. Indeed, even other cytokines not originally identified by their effects on hematopoietic cells, such as tumor necrosis factor (TNF) and transforming growth factor-beta (TGF-β) have important regulatory effects on hematopoiesis. In humans, a rise in TNF levels often precedes graft versus host disease (GVHD), and the severity of GVHD has been observed to correlate with TNF levels.

Besides the importance of cytokines in understanding cell growth, differentiation, and division, their production has made some of them available for treatment purposes. To date, the most notable of this class of compounds have been α-interferon, currently widely used in the treatment of chronic leukemias; various marrow stimulatory factors (granulocyte colony-stimulating factor [G-CSF], thrombopoietin [TPO], interleukin-3 [IL3], and others); and the immunostimulatory leukokines—notably IL2 and the differentiating vitamins, the most notable to date being all-transretinoic acid (ATRA) with its dramatic and mechanistically defined effect on malignant promyelocytes. Table 6.1 depicts the growth factors, their cell source, and their functions as they are currently known at the time of this writing. This

Table 6.1
Growth Factors

Cytokines	Cell Sources	Functions
IL1	Monocytes-macrophages B cells Epithelial cells Fibroblasts, astrocytes Dendritic cells Keratinocytes	Endogenous pyrogen Growth factor for lymphocytes, fibroblasts, synovial cells, endothelial cells, hematopoietic cells Induction of acute-phase proteins
IL2	Activated T cells	Growth and differentiation factor for lymphocytes and endothelial cells
IL3, G-CSF, GM-CSF, M-CSF	Monocytes, T cells	Growth factors for hematopoietic cells
IL4	Activated T-cells	Growth and differentiation factor for lymphocytes
IL5	T cells	Eosinophil growth factor, B-cell differentiation factor
IL6	Monocytes-macrophages B cells Epithelial cells Fibroblasts, astrocytes Dendritic cells Keratinocytes	Endogenous pyrogen Growth factor for lymphocytes, fibroblasts, synovial cells, endothelial cells, hematopoietic cells Induction of acute phase proteins Plasma cell growth factor
IL7	Bone marrow stroma cells Spleen cells	Growth factor of pre-B and pre-T lymphocytes
IL8	Monocytes T lymphocytes	Neutrophil chemotactic factor
IL9	T lymphocytes	T-cell growth factor
IL10	T lymphocytes	T-helper cell inhibitory factor Stem cell growth factor
IL11	Stromal cells	Multifunctional regulator of hematopoiesis

(Continued)

Table 6.1   (*Continued*)

Cytokines	Cell Sources	Functions
IL12	Human B lymphoblastoid cell line (NC-37)	Functional activation of NK cells Induction of LAK cells synergistically with IL2 Augmentation of allogeneic CTL response Enhancement of IL2-induced proliferation of resting peripheral blood cells
IL13	Th 2 cells	Induces proliferation, Ig isotype switching, and Ig synthesis Down modulates macrophage activity Induces IgE synthesis
IL14	T cells Some malignant B cells	Induces B-cell proliferation Inhibits immunoglobulin secretion Selectively expands certain B-cell populations
IL15	Epithelial and fibroblast cell lines Adherent peripheral blood mononuclear cells	Stimulates proliferation of IL2-dependent cell line and activated peripheral blood T cells Induces generation of cytolytic effector cells in vitro
IL16	Eosinophils	Chemoattractant or lymphocytes (CD4+) and eosinophils Induces rapid translocation of protein kinase C from the cytosol to the membrane in CD4+ cells
IL17	Activated memory CD4+ T cells	Early initiator of T cell-dependent inflammatory reaction Element of cytokine network that bridges the immune system to hematopoiesis

(Continued)

Table 6.1   (Continued)

Cytokines	Cell Sources	Functions
IL18	Liver cells	Interferon-gamma (IFN-γ) inducing factor IFN-γ production by spleen Enhancement of NK cytotoxicity Augments GM-CSF production Decreases IL10 production
IFN-α	Buffy coat leukocytes Namaliva cells KG1 cells Akube cells B lymphocytes CML cells Fibroblasts induced by viruses	Inhibition of growth of tumor cells Stimulation of NK cell activity Stimulation of cytotoxic T cells and macrophages
IFNβ	Fibroblasts Some epithelial cells, such as amniotic cells Osteosarcoma MG63 Embryonic tissue Breast carcinosarcoma	Increases cell surface Cell surface HLA class I and II antigen Serum B_2-microglobulin Serum neopterin NK activity Lymphocyte CD38 reactivity 2,5 a synthetase activity in peripheral blood lymphocytes Antibody-dependent cellular cytotoxicity
IFNγ	T and NK cells	Antiviral activity antiproliferative activity on tumor cells Induction of MHC class I and II antigens Activates macrophages to become tumoricidal and kill intracellular parasites Enhances NK cell activity

(Continued)

Table 6.1 *(Continued)*

Cytokines	Cell Sources	Functions
		Induces immunoglobulin secretion by B cells and enhances B-cell motivation and proliferation
		Inhibits osteoclast activation
Interferon (IFN)	T and NK cells	Differentiation factor for B cells
		Activator of NK cells and macrophages
Tumor necrosis factor (TNF) α/β	Monocytes T cells	Antivirus
		Cytotoxic factor
		Cachectin
		Septic shock
		Growth factor for hematopoietic and fibroblastic cells
Thrombopoietin (TPO)	Kidney, liver, bone marrow, spleen	Regulation of platelet production

From: Friedman WH. Pathophysiology of cytokines. Leuk Res 1990;14(8):675–677. Pumonen PJ, deVries JE. IL13 induces proliferation, Ig isotype switching, and Ig synthesis by immature human fetal B cells. J Immunol 1994;152:1094–1102. Ambrus JL Jr, Pippin J, Joseph A, et al. Identification of cDNA for a human high-molecular weight B-cell growth factor. Proc Natl Acad Sci USA 1993;90:6330–6334. Grabstein KH, Eisenman J, Shanebeck K, et al. Cloning of a T cell growth factor that interacts with the B chain of the interleukin-2 receptor. Science 1994;264:965–968. Lim KG, Wan HC, Bozza PT, et al. Human eosinophils elaborate the lymphocyte chemoattractants. IL16 (lymphocyte chemoattractant factor) and RANTES. J Immunol 1996;156(7):2566–2570. Fossiez F, Djossou O, Chomarat P, et al. T cell interleukin-17 induces stromal cells to produce proinflammatory and hematopoietic cytokines. J Exp Med 1996;183(6):2593–2603. Ushio S, Namba M, Okura T, et al. Cloning of the cDNA for human IFN-gamma-inducing factor, expression in Escherichia coli, and studies on the biologic activities of the protein. J Immunol 1996;156(11):4274–4279. Sungaran R, Markovic B, Chong BH. Localization and regulation of thrombopoietin mRNA expression in human kidney, liver, bone marrow and spleen using in situ hybridization. Blood 1997;89:101–107.

will undoubtedly change rapidly as this burgeoning field expands into the future. The cytokines are discussed in this chapter in relation to diagnosis and classification of the acute leukemias that have presented unique, unusual, and controversial problems. Table 6.2 shows the difficult and controversial leukemias in relation to cytokines with comments and references.

ACUTE UNDIFFERENTIATED LEUKEMIA (AUL)

As technology advances, the number of cases of AUL seen will become progressively smaller; however, Meckenstock et al. studied a case of AUL by surface marker analysis using two color immunofluorescence staining. The blast cells expressed CD34, CD38, CD117, and class II antigens. The cells coexpressed TdT, CD4, CD7, CD13, CD19, and CD22. Cytoplasmic expression of myeloperoxidase, CD3, and CD22 could not be demonstrated.

Table 6.2
Summary of Cytokines

Diagnosis FAB Subtype	Cytokines	Comment	References
Acute undifferentiated leukemia (AUL)	AUL blast cells showed increased DNA synthesis with IL3, IL6, and G-CSF in vitro	Presence of functional GM-CSF receptors on AUL blast cells has clinical implications	Leukemia 1995;9:260–264 Int J Cell Cloning 1992;10:166–172
Hypocellular/ aplastic ALL	No data available on these disorders. Traditional ALL blast cells rarely respond to growth factors	Growth factors have greater influence on AML blasts than ALL blasts	Leukemia 1993;7:1026–1033
Granular ALL	Rare case of T-granular ALL reported with increase in TGF-beta 1, IL2, IL2R, IL6, IL8	Need more cases with cytokines studied to make any conclusions	Am J Hematol 1995;49:349–352
ALL with eosinophilia	IL3, IL5, and GM-CSF secreted by malignant cells. Eosinophila associated with B-lineage ALL t(5;14)	Eosinophils are part of neoplastic process in FAB M4Eo, FAB M2t(8;21), CML. Contrariwise, eosinophils are reactive in ALL t(5;14), malignant lymphoma, Hodgkin lymphoma, and adult T-cell lymphoma/ leukemia	Genes Chrom Cancer 1993;8:219–223 Nippon Rinsho 1993;51:800–805
ALL t(4;11)	IL4 used as apoptotic agent that shows promise for use in clinical trials on high risk ALLs resistant to conventional therapy	Additional studies needed in area of cytokines to better treat high-risk patients	Blood 1994;83:1731–1737
ALL-hand mirror variant	No studies of cytokines performed on hand mirror cases	Formation of HMV related to immune complexes to BaEV in part. Recent studies have described mixed leukemias and adhesive molecules. Data not clear	Am J Clin Pathol 1992;98:526–530 Hematopathol Mol Hematol 1996;10: 85–98
Aggressive NK cell leukemia (ANKCL)	NK cells in culture dependent on IL2 not other cytokines	Established NK cell line source for studies of NK cell biology	Exp Hematol 1996;24:406–415
AML-M0	Kasumi-3 cell line (FAB AML M0) shows high level *EVI* 1 gene expression. Kasumi-3 cells proliferate when exposed to either IL2, IL3, IL4, GM-CSF, or stem cell factor	Cell line helpful in studying FAB AML M0 and investigating role of *EVI*-1 gene in leukemogenesis	JAP J Cancer Res 1996;87:269–274

(Continued)

Table 6.2 *(Continued)*

Diagnosis FAB Subtype	Cytokines	Comment	References
AML-M6 erythroleukemia	GM-CSF, IL3, IL4, IL5, IL13, and stem cell factor stimulates erythroleukemia cell line TF1	Studies on cell lines give insights into growth control of various cytokines	Blood 1995;86:2534–2540 Blood 1995;86:2679–2688 FEBS letters 1995;366:122–126
Acute basophilic leukemia	ber/abl encoded proteins and IL3 enhance basophilic differentiation. Tyrosine kinases involved in activation signal of human basophils	Tyrosine phosphorylation activated in part by hematopoietic cytokines, especially IL3. Links growth factor receptors to gene transcription	J Exp Med 1996;183:811–820 J Leukocyte Biol 1996;59:461–470
Eosinophilic leukemia/ hypereosinophilic syndrome	Eosinophilia in hematologic malignancies may be due to chromosomes, cytokines or both. Cytokines that stimulate eosinophilia include GM-CSF, IL1, IL3, IL5	Pathology related to eosinophilic granules which may produce similar disease in EL and HES.	Cancer Genet Cytogenet 1995;83:37–41 Acta Haematologica 1995;88:207–212
Hypocellular AML	Increased cytokines (IL1, IL6, TNF-alpha) may be a reactive response in hypocellular bone marrow	Cytokine studies performed on aplastic anemia, MDS and various leukemias, but not hypocellular bone marrow	Leuk Res 1995;19:639–644 Exp Hematol 1993;21:80–85
CD7 positive AML	CD7 AML cell line (HSM911) responds to rGM-CSF, rIL3, and rSCF	HSM911 may be useful cell line for studying CD7 AML	Hokkaido J Med Science 1994;69:750–766
AML inv 3(q21;q26)	No cytokine data on AML inv 3(q21;q26)	Studies on other AMLs have determined that IL9 may play a role in AML	Blood 1996;87:3852–3859
Myeloid/NK leukemia	NK cells are source of IL3 and GM-CSF	IL3 and GM-CSF may act as autocrine growth factors in this leukemia. Cytokines that induce NK cell IF-γ cause apoptosis of NK cells	Stem Cells 1995;13:324–335 Blood 1997;89:910–918
Bilineage/biphenotypic acute leukemia	Heterogeneity of response by bilineal and biphenotypic leukemias to cytokines	FLT3R expressed by most (80 to 100%) of mixed-lineage leukemias	Leukemia 1996;10:588–599

Also, absence of clonal rearrangements of immunoglobulin or T-cell receptor genes was shown by Southern blot analysis. Of interest was the observation that DNA synthesis of the leukemic blasts measured by ^{3}H-thymidine could be stimulated by IL3, IL6, and G-CSF in vitro. The authors speculated that the leukemic cells represented an early, most immature developmental stage within a multipotent progenitor cell compartment. Tsao et al. examined the stimulatory effects of recombinant human GM-CSF and IL6 on the in vitro proliferation of leukemic blast cells from patients with acute leukemia. The GM-CSF stimulated DNA synthesis of blast cells in 9 of 14 (64%) AML cases, two cases of AUL, and one case of acute mixed leukemia. Only two cases of AML blasts responded to IL6 as demonstrated by growth in short-term suspension cultures. GM-CSF and IL6 did not display a synergistic effect on the growth of leukemic cells. Of importance was the finding by the authors that the leukemic blast cells of AUL and acute mixed leukemia possessed functional GM-CSF receptors. Such a finding has clear clinical implications and suggests that growth factors may be deleterious in some leukemias.

ACUTE LYMPHOBLASTIC LEUKEMIA (ALL)

Hypocellular/Aplastic ALL

The hypocellular/aplastic ALLs have not been evaluated for cytokines. The acellular nature of these disorders would suggest that cell growth, proliferation, and division are operating under different control mechanisms than traditional cases of ALL. Indeed, the hypocellular/aplastic event is typically followed by apparent bone marrow recovery and later by overt leukemia in a matter of weeks or a few months. Mirro et al. evaluated blast cells from 52 cases of pediatric AML and 81 cases of ALL to 11 hematopoietic growth factors by ^{3}H-thymidine assay. Blasts from almost one half of the patients (25 out of 52) with AML responded to growth factors such as IL3, G-CSF, or GM-CSF. Alternatively, 37% of AML cases (19 out of 52) showed little thymidine incorporation in the presence of growth factors and were classified as nonresponsive. In striking contrast to the AML cases, blast cells from only a few of the ALL cases studied showed any response to growth factors. Such results demonstrate that growth factor responsiveness is a unique biological characteristic of the leukemic blasts and does not appear to correlate with other identified biological features.

Granular ALL

Little information is present in the literature on cytokines and ALL with cytoplasmic granules. Dalal et al. investigated a case of aggressive large granular lymphocytic leukemia with acute myelofibrosis. The leukemic cells were immature T-cells (CD5+, CD7+, CD16−, CD56−, CD57−,

CD41−), with a monosomy 7. They secreted large amounts of TGF-β 1. The serum levels of IL2, IL2R, IL6, and IL8 were elevated, while the IL1-β, IL4, and TNF-α were normal.

ALL with Eosinophilia

Eosinophilia in hematological malignancies may be in relation to chromosomal changes or cytokine production. In some myelogenous leukemias, including acute myelomonocytic leukemia with eosinophilia (FAB AML M4Eo), acute myeloblastic leukemia [FAB AML M2 t(8;21)] and chronic myelogenous leukemia, neoplastic cells themselves appear to differentiate into eosinophils. On the other hand, transformed tumor cells secrete some eosinophil-stimulating cytokines, including IL3, IL5, and GM-CSF. These cytokines stimulate the proliferation of normal eosinophil precursors in some lymphoid malignancies, including some types of B-lineage ALL (especially with t(5;14) or malignant lymphoma, including Hodgkin's lymphoma and adult T-cell lymphoma/leukemia). Knuutila et al. applied the morphology-antibody-chromosomic technique to samples of the bone marrow and cerebrospinal fluid in a patient with ALL, eosinophilia, and a 5;14 translocation. The karyotype of the blast cells was 47, XY, +X, t(5;14)(q31;q32), I(7) q(10). Interphase cytogenetic study by in situ hybridization with a X-specific alphoid probe revealed the abnormality in CD10, CD19, and TdT positive lymphoid cells, whereas CD13 positive, Sudan black B positive, eosinophilic, and basophilic granulocytes, as well as monocytes and small lymphocytes did not demonstrate the abnormality. Such results clearly show that eosinophils do not belong to the malignant clone, but are reactive. Of interest at the molecular level is that B-lineage ALL with eosinophilia and the t(5;14)(q31;q32) demonstrate involvement of the IgH gene and IL3 gene. Activation of the IL3 gene results in cytokine release partly responsible for the eosinophilia observed in these cases.

ALL t(4;11)

Manabe et al. have observed that IL4 induces programmed cell death (apoptosis) in cases of high-risk ALL. They evaluated the survival of leukemic and normal B-cell progenitors cultured on bone marrow stroma. IL4 was cytotoxic in 16 of 21 cases of B-lineage ALL, causing reductions in CD19+ cell numbers that ranged from 50% to greater than 99% of those in parallel cultures not exposed to the cytokine. All nine cases with t(4;11)(q21;q23) or t(9;22)(q34;q11), chromosomal features that are often associated with multidrug resistance and a fatal outcome, were susceptible to IL4 toxicity. The IL4 cytotoxicity resulted from induction of programmed cell death (apoptosis), and there was no evidence of cell killing mediated by T, natural killer, or stromal cells. Also, IL4 cytotoxicity extended to a proportion of normal

B-cell progenitors. Nevertheless, the authors felt that clinical testing of IL4 in cases of high risk lymphoblastic leukemia, e.g., t(4;11) resistant to conventional therapy, is indicated.

ALL-Hand Mirror Variant (HMV)

Factors controlling the formation of hand mirror cells (HMCs) in ALL are not completely understood. It has been shown that antigen, antigen-antibody complexes, anti-Ig, phytohemagglutinin, and a wide variety of immunological reactions mediated by the Fc receptor can induce human lymphocytes to form HMCs.

Investigation of bone marrow plasma has shown immune complexes to the baboon endogenous virus (BaEV). Two patients studied in detail by Western blot analysis revealed cross reactive IgG to the envelope gp70 and IgM against core p30 proteins of BaEV and the Simian sarcoma associated virus (SSAV). Also, IgM antibodies to the gp70 were observed in the ALL-HMV, but not other non-hand mirror leukemic patients or the normal controls. Furthermore, immunoperoxidase tagged IgM antibodies prepared from the first patient's bone marrow with ALL-HMV reacted with her own HMC and revealed BaEV antigen on the tip of the uropod. The significance of these findings remains unclear. Recent studies have shown that some ALL-HMVs demonstrate mixed lineage and adhesion molecules on their surface. No studies have been performed to evaluate cytokines. Additional studies are needed to clarify the nature of this heterogeneous group of disorders.

AGGRESSIVE NATURAL KILLER CELL LEUKEMIA (ANKCL)

Robertson et al. have successfully established a cell line from the peripheral blood from a patient with an ANKCL. The immunophenotype revealed CD3−, CD16+, CD56+ large granular lymphocytes. The morphology of the natural killer (NK) cells resembled that of normal activated NK cells. The neoplastic cells mediated natural killing, antibody-dependent cellular cytotoxicity, and exhibited proliferative responses similar to normal CD16+ CD56 dim NK cells. These NK cells were strictly dependent on IL2 for sustained growth and die if deprived of IL2 for more than 7 days. NK cells growing in the presence of IL2 express abundant IL2R-α with little or no detectable IL2-β or γ chain on the cell surface. NK cells deprived of IL2 express high levels of both IL2R-α and β. IL4, IL7, and IL12, unlike IL2, do not maintain viability of the NK cells. Furthermore, IL1, IL4, IL6, IL7, IL12, TNF-α, interferon-alpha (INF-α), and IFN-γ do not support the growth of the NK cells. The authors state that the NK cell line may prove useful for studies of human NK cell biology.

ACUTE MYELOID LEUKEMIA (AML)

AML M0

Asou et al. have developed a novel human leukemia cell line (Kasumi-3) that was established from the blast cells of a 57-year-old man suffering from myeloperoxidase-negative acute leukemia (FAB AML M0). Flow cytometric analyses revealed cell surface expression of CD7, CD4, CD13, CD33, CD34, HLA-DR, and c-Kit. Karyotypic studies showed t(3;7)(q27:q22), del(5)(q15), del (9)(q32), and add (12)(p11). The breakpoint 3q27 was located near the *EVI* 1 gene, and a high level of expression of the *EVI* 1 gene was observed. Treatment with either IL2, IL3, IL4, GM-CSF, or stem cell factor (SCF) induced the proliferation of Kasumi-3 cells. Therefore, the Kasumi-3 cell line shows the characteristic features of undifferentiated leukemia (FAB AML M0). Such a cell line should be useful for studying the biological characteristics of FAB AML M0 and for investigating the role of the *EVI* 1 gene in leukemogenesis.

AML M6-Erythroleukemia

Most studies of cytokines in erythroleukemia have been limited to leukemic cell lines. Mire-Sluis et al. investigated a human erythroleukemia cell line, TF-1, and demonstrated that it proliferates in response to GM-CSF, IL3, and IL5. Interestingly they found that each cytokine had a specific alpha unit, but all three share a common beta chain. Also, they determined that GM-CSF and IL3 use tyrosine phosphorylation to mediate mitogenic signal transduction; whereas, IL5 uses tyrosine dephosphorylation. The authors suggested that since these cytokines share the identical beta chain of their receptors, the cytokine specific alpha chain mediates the linkage to each receptor to the individual biochemical signal transduction pathways responsible for the different biologic activities of these cytokines. In addition, Lefort et al. found that IL13 and IL4 are growth factors for the erythroleukemia TF-1 cell line. Furthermore, Pietsch demonstrated significant response to SCF with cell lines of acute promyelocytic, chronic myeloid, megakaryoblastic, and erythroleukemic origin. Moreover, by using PCR analysis of total RNA from the myeloid leukemia cell lines, he found expression of SCF mRNA in 17 of 30 cell lines, suggesting autocrine mechanisms in the growth of a subgroup of leukemic cells by coexpression of SCF and its receptor.

Acute Basophilic Leukemia (ABL)

Human basophils are activated through high-affinity immunoglobulin E(Ig E) receptors (Fc epsilon RI) and are involved in late phase of the allergic reaction. Interestingly, only acute basophilic leukemic cells expressed Fc epsilon RI. Aggregation of Fc epsilon RI by IgE and anti-IgE, IgE and antigen, or anti-Fc epsilon RI monoclonal antibodies on ABL cells led to increased tyrosine phosphorylation. Benhamou et al. performed studies that indicated that these tyrosine kinases are involved in the early steps of human Fc epsilon signaling in basophils. Carlesso et al. studied tyrosyl phosphorylation and DNA binding activity of signal transducers and activators of transcription (STAT) proteins in hematopoietic cell lines transformed by bcr/abl. They observed that some of the biological effects of bcr/abl overlap with those of hematopoietic cytokines, particularly IL3. These effects included mitogenesis, enhanced survival, and enhanced basophilic differentiation. Therefore, it has been suggested that p210 $^{bcr/abl}$ and the IL3 receptor may activate some common signal transduction pathway. An important pathway for IL3 signaling involves activation of the Janus family kinases and subsequent tyrosyl phosphorylation of STAT. This pathway directly links growth factor receptors to gene transcription.

Eosinophilic Leukemia (EL)/Hypereosinophilic Syndrome (HES)

Hematological malignancies accompanied by eosinophilia may occur in relation to chromosomal change, cytokine production, or both. Eosinophilia, accompanied by hematological malignancies, can be divided into two groups. In some myelogenous leukemias, including acute myelomonocytic leukemia with eosinophilia (FAB AML M4Eo), acute myeloblastic leukemia [FAB AML M2 t(8;21)], and chronic myelogenous leukemia, neoplastic cells themselves appear to differentiate into eosinophils. Contrariwise, transformed tumor cells secrete some eosinophil-stimulating-cytokines including IL3, IL5, and GM-CSF. These cytokines stimulate the proliferation of normal eosinophil precursors in some lymphoid malignancies, including some types of ALL (especially t(5;14) or malignant lymphoma, including Hodgkin's disease and adult T cell lymphoma/leukemia). Apparently, the eosinophilia in the HES is related to production of soluble eosinopoietic factors including IL5 by T lymphocytes. Abe et al. have reported a case of FAB AML M2 in which the number of leukemic clones with additional abnormalities of chromosome 5 increased with concurrent development of eosinophilia, fever, asthmalike symptoms erythema, itching, and hepatosplenomegaly. The authors postulated that the increase in IL5 may have been produced by an abnormality on chromosome 5. Such a finding would implicate a chromosomal abnormality that induced increased cytokine production.

Hypocellular AML

Little is written on hypocellular AML and cytokines; however, Koike et al. have evaluated cytokine production by peripheral blood mononuclear cells in patients with aplastic anemia and myelodysplastic syndromes. The levels of IL6, IL1-β, and tissue necrosis factor-α were markedly elevated in aplastic anemia and refractory anemia. The levels were not as high in refractory anemia with excess blasts (RAEB) or refractory anemia with excess blasts in transformation (RAEB-IT). The authors observed high cytokine levels in hypocellular marrows in association with low blast counts. They suggested that the increased cytokines may be a reactive response in hypocellular bone marrow. Unfortunately, the authors did not study any patients with hypocellular AML.

Kurzrock et al. evaluated a number of patients with acute and chronic leukemia for expression of IL1-β and TNF-α. TNF-α was discerned in almost half of the samples 27 (47%), and was expressed in some patients with every type of leukemia, except T-cell ALL. Expression occurred with great frequency in samples (12 of 15 [80%]) from monocytic (acute or chronic) leukemias and from advanced CLL. IL1-β transcripts were detected in 20 of 57 samples (35%). Its presence, like TNF-α, was ubiquitous, and only CLL and T-cell ALL cells consistently failed to produce IL1-β message. The authors postulated that the widespread constitutive expression by neoplastic blood cells may play a fundamental role in driving the leukemic process.

CD7 positive AML

Iwasaki has studied a novel CD7-positive leukemia cell line (HSM911) derived from the peripheral blood of a patient with AML. Proliferation assay using a variety of cytokines demonstrated that the HSM911 cells proliferate in response to recombinant GM-CSF (rGM-CSF), recombinant IL3 (rIL3), and recombinant SCF (rSCF), but do not respond to recombinant G-CSF (rG-CSF), natural macrophage CSF (M-CSF), rIL1, rIL2, rIL4, rIL5, rIL, or recombinant erythropoietin. Interestingly, polyclonal anti GM-CSF and polyclonal anti-IL3 antibody blocked the proliferation of HSM911 stimulated with rGM-CSF and rIL3. HSM911 maintained in the presence of rGM-CSF expressed the CD7, CD13, CD33, CD34, LCD41a, HLA-DR, VLA1-VLA5, CD11a, CD54, CD44, and LAM 1. These findings suggest that HSM911 might be of multipotent progenitor cell origin. The author expressed that HSM911 is a useful tool for analyzing CD7-positive AML. Also, such studies could possibly provide useful therapeutic information.

AML inv 3(q21;q26)

Cytokine studies on this variant of AML have not been reported in the literature; however, as mentioned previously, various cytokines have been evaluated in AML on cell lines. In addition, Lemoli et al. have evaluated the proliferative response of 32 primary samples from AML patients to recombinant human IL9 alone and combined with recombinant human IL3, GM-CSF, and SCF. They determined that IL9 may play a role in the development of AML by stimulating leukemic cells to enter the S-phase rather than preventing cell death. Moreover, they found that IL9 acts synergistically with SCF for recruiting quiescent leukemic cells in cell cycle.

The effects of cytokines on leukemic and normal hematopoietic cells is a burgeoning area of hematologic research. It represents an area that will give us increased insights and understanding of normal hematopoiesis and leukemogenesis.

Myeloid/NK Leukemia

This unique acute leukemic variant first reported by Scott et al. showed the unusual immunophenotype: CD33+, CD56+, CD11a+, CD13lo, CD15lo, CD34+/-, HLA-DR-, and CD16-. These cases demonstrated morphologic and cytochemical findings remarkably similar to those of acute promyelocytic leukemia. The authors did not study growth factors or cytokines in this exclusive group.

Recently Nimer and Uchida have studied regulation of GM-CSF and IL3 expression. These cytokines are multilineage acting hematopoietic growth factors that have overlapping but distinct biological properties. Cellular sources of IL3 are confined to activated T cells, NK cells, mast cells, and, possibly, megakaryocytes, while these cells and activated macrophages, fibroblasts, and endothelial cells are important sources of GM-CSF. Interestingly, in vitro studies have implicated both cytokines in the autocrine growth of human myeloid or murine mast cell lines. Since NK cells are a source of IL3, future studies of cytokines on myeloid/NK acute leukemia would seem indicated.

Most recently, Ross and Coligiuri have demonstrated that cytokines induce apoptosis in NK cells. Interferon-γ (IFN-γ) is critical for an effective innate immune response against infection. A combination of interleukins derived from activated T cells (IL2) and monocytes (IL12), or monocytes alone (IL15 and IL12) induces optimal production of IFN-γ from natural killer cells. The authors showed that the cytokines that induce NK cell IF-γ production subsequently induce apoptosis of the NK cells. They propose that this novel observation may have implications for the regulation of the innate immune response during infection, the toxicity of combination cytokine therapy, and the treatment of NK cell leukemia. The latter utilization would add a new and exciting role to the use of cytokines in the leukemias.

BILINEAGE/BIPHENOTYPIC ACUTE LEUKEMIA

Investigation of cytokines in bilineage/biphenotypic acute leukemia has been limited in the literature. Nevertheless, Kita et al. have studied two patients with CML mixed crisis and one with Ph[1] ALL with cross lineage. These cases demonstrated a considerable number of granulocytes with monoclonally rearranged immunogenotype. In a colony assay of cells from the Ph[1] ALL patients, the leukemic cells showed the potential to differentiate into granulocytes in the presence of either GM-CSF or G-CSF. Interleukin 7 exerted synergistic effects on colony and cluster formation in cultures with these cytokines. Furthermore, IL3, GM-CSF and G-CSF receptor gene expression was found in the leukemic cells. The authors indicated that the Ph[1] + common progenitors in the three cases preserved the potential for granulocytic differentiation even after the occurrence of the Ig and TCR gene rearrangements as the first genomic event in lymphocyte differentiation. Also, Tsao et al. observed specific binding of GM-CSF on blast cells of acute mixed-lineage leukemia and AUL.

Contrariwise, Hassan et al. have studied a new CD34+ human multilineage myeloid leukemia cell line MHH225. This multipotent myeloid leukemic clone contained a mixed population of megakaryoblastic, erythroblastic, and myeloblastic cells in a serum-free culture. Surprisingly, none of the myelopoietic growth factors, i.e., IL3, GM-CSF, GSF, erythropoietin, or IL6 had any effect on the proliferation and/or differentiation of the MHH 25 cells. The authors offered no explanation for lack of response, but stated that the MHH25 cell line is the first human CD34+ leukemia cell line growing in serum-free cultures to be established.

Recently, Drexler has studied the novel hematopoietic growth factor FLT3 ligand. This ligand is the cognate ligand for the FLT3, tyrosine kinase receptor (R), also referred to as FLK-2 and STK-1. The FLT3R belongs to a family of receptor tyrosine kinases involved in hematopoiesis that also includes KIT, the receptor for SCF. At the mRNA level FLT3R was expressed by most cases (80 to 100%) of acute mixed-lineage leukemia, AML, ALL, and CML in lymphoid or mixed blast crisis. The author noted that such findings further underlined the heterogeneity of various leukemic samples in their proliferative response to cytokine.

BIBLIOGRAPHY

Articles

Abe A, Tanimoto M, Towatari M, et al. Acute myeloblastic leukemia (M2) with translocation (7;11) followed by marked eosinophilia and additional abnormalities of chromosome 5. Can Genet Cytogenet 1995;83:37–41.

Asou H, Suzukawa K, Kita K, et al. Establishment of an undifferentiated leukemia cell line (Kasumi-3) with t(3;7) (q27;q22) and activation of the EVI 1 gene. Jap J Cancer Res 1996;87(3):269–274.

Bellone G, Trinchieri G. Dual stimulatory and inhibitory effect of NK cell stimulatory factor/IL-12 on human hematopoiesis. J Immunol 1994;153:930–937.

Benhamou M, Feuillard J, Lortholary O, et al. Protein tyrosine kinases in activation signal of human basophils through the immunoglobulin E receptor type 1. J Leukoc Biol 1996;59(3):416–470.

Carlesso N, Frank DA, Griffin JD. Tyrosyl phosphorylation and DNA binding activity of signal transducers and activators of transcription (STAT) proteins in hematopoietic cell lines transformed by bcr/abl. J Exp Med 1996;183:811–820.

Cherel M, Sorel M, LeBeau B, et al. Molecular cloning of two isoforms of a receptor for the human hematopoietic cytokine interleukin-11. Blood 1995;86(7):2534–2540.

Dalal BI, Keown PA, Paraskevas F, et al. Cytokine profile in acute myelofibrosis associated with aggressive large granular lymphocyte leukemia. Am J Hematol 1995;49(4):349–352.

Fossiez F, Djossou O, Chomarat P, et al. T cell interleukin-17 induces stromal cells to produce proinflammatory and hematopoietic cytokines. J Exp Med 1996; 183:2593–2603.

Hassan HT, Petershofen E, Lux E, et al. Establishment and characterization of a novel CD34-positive human myeloid leukemia cell line: MHH225 growing in serum-free culture. Ann Hematol 1995;71:111–117.

Iwasaki H. Cellular and biological characterization of CD7-positive acute leukemia cells—an investigation of the established cell line, HSM911. Hokkaido J Med Sci 1994;69:750–766.

Kita K, Shimizu N, Miwa H, et al. A granulocytic population with rearranged immunogenotype in chronic myelocytic leukemia blast crisis and Philadelphia-chromosome-positive acute leukemia with cross-lineage nature. Leukemia 1993;7(2):251–257.

Knuutila S, Alitalo R, Ruutu T. Power of the MAC (morphology-antibody-chromosomes) method in distinguishing reactive and clonal cells: report of a patient with acute lymphatic leukemia, eosinophilia and t(5;14). Genes Chromosom Cancer 1993;8(4):219–223.

Koike M, Ishiyama T, Tomoyasu S, et al. Spontaneous cytokine overproduction by peripheral blood mononuclear cells from patients with myelodysplastic syndromes and aplastic anemia. Leuk Res 1995;19:639–644.

Kovarik P, Shrit MA, Yuen B, et al. Hand mirror variant of acute lymphoblastic leukemia. Evidence for a mixed leukemia. Am J Clin Pathol 1992;98:526–530.

Kurzrock R, Kantarjian H, Wetzler M, et al. Ubiquitous expression of cytokines in diverse leukemias of lymphoid and myeloid lineage. Exp Hematol 1993;21:80–85.

Lefort S, Vita N, Reeb R, et al. IL-13 and IL-4 share signal transduction elements as well as receptor components in TF-1 cells. FEBS Lett 1995;366(2-3):122–126.

Lemoli RM, Fortuna A, Tafuri A, et al. Interleukin-9 stimulates the proliferation of human myeloid leukemic cells. Blood 1996;87:3852–3859.

Lim KG, Wan HC, Bozza PT, et al. Human eosinophils elaborate the lymphocyte chemoattractants. IL-16 (lymphocyte chemoattractant factor) and RANTES. J Immunol 1996;156(7):2566–2570.

Manabe A, Coustan-Smith E, Kumagai M, et al. Interleukin-4 induces programmed cell death (apoptosis) in cases of high-risk acute lymphoblastic leukemia. Blood 1994;83(7):1731–1737.

Meckenstock G, Heyll A, Schneider EM, et al. Acute leukemia coexpressing myeloid, B- and T-lineage associated markers: multiparameter analysis of criteria defining lineage commitment and maturational stage in a case of undifferentiated leukemia. Leukemia 1995;9(2):260–264.

Mire-Sluis A, Page LA, Wadhwa M, et al. Evidence for a signaling role for the alpha chains of granulocyte-macrophage colony-stimulating factor (GM-CSF) interleukin-3 (IL-3), and IL-5 receptors: divergent signaling pathways between GM-CSF/IL-3 and IL-5. Blood 1995;86(7):2679–2688.

Mirro J Jr, Hurwitz CA, Behm FG, et al. Effects of recombinant human hematopoietic growth factors on leukemic blasts from children with acute myeloblastic or lymphoblastic leukemia. Leukemia 1993;7(7):1026–1033.

Pietsch T. Paracrine and autocrine growth mechanisms of human stem cell factor (c-kit ligand) in myeloid leukemia. Nouv Rev Fr Hematol 1993;35(3):285–286.

Robertson MJ, Cochran KJ, Cameron C, et al. Characterization of a cell line, NKL, derived from an aggressive human natural killer cell leukemia. Exp Hematol 1996;24(3):406–415.

Ross ME, Coligiuri MA. Cytokine-induced apoptosis of human natural killer cells identifies a novel mechanism to regulate the innate immune response. Blood 1997;89:910–918.

Schumacher HR, Desai SN, McClain KL, et al. Acute lymphoblastic leukemia-hand mirror variant. Analysis for endogenous retroviral antibodies in bone marrow plasma Am J Clin Pathol 1989;91:410–416.

Scott AA, Head DR, Kopecky KJ, et al. HLA-DR–, CD33+, CD56+, CD16– myeloid/natural killer cell acute leukemia: a previously unrecognized form of acute leukemia potentially misdiagnosed as French-American-British acute myeloid leukemia-M3. Blood 1994;84:244–255.

Tsao CJ, Cheng TY, Chang SL, et al. Effects of granulocyte-macrophage colony-stimulating factor and interleukin 6 on the growth of leukemic blasts in suspension culture. Int J Cell Cloning 1992;10(3):166–172.

Ushio S, Namba M, Okura T, et al. Cloning of the cDNA for human IFN-gamma-inducing factor, expression in Escherichia coli, and studies on the biologic activities of the protein. J Immunol 1996;156:4274–4279.

Wibowo A, Pankowsky D, Mikhael A, et al. Adult acute leukemia: hand mirror cell variant. Hematopathol Mol Hematol 1996;10:85–98.

Yano A, Yasukawa M, Yanagisawa K, et al. Adult T cell leukemia associated with eosinophilia: analysis of eosinophil-stimulating factors produced by leukemic cells. Acta Haematologica 1992;88:207–212.

Review Articles

Drexler HG. Expression of FLT3 receptor and response to FLT3 ligand by leukemic cells. Leukemia 1996;10:588–599.

Nimer SD, Uchida H. Regulation of granulocyte-macrophage colony-stimulating factor and interleukin 3 expression. Stem Cells 1995;13:324–335.

Okamura S, Ikematsu W. Hematological malignancies with eosinophilia. Nippon Rinsho 1993;51:800–805.

CHAPTER 7

The Automated Leukocyte Count and Differential: The Future Approach to Diagnosis

GENERAL COMMENTS

The purpose of this chapter is to provide a brief history of automated flow leukocyte counting and differentiation, plus an understanding of how to-day's automated flow leukocyte count and differential are generated and may be used to detect acute leukemia.

Today, automated instrumentation is the mainstay of the routine hematology laboratory. This is because it is no longer possible, with the staffing available, to use manual methods to meet the ever-increasing demand for screening slides, accurate differentials, follow-up blood counts and precise diagnosis. In addition, automating pipetting, diluting, and counting large numbers of cells increases accuracy and precision.

Cells counted and differentiated in suspension are random events that follow a Poisson distribution for the count and standard error of proportion (SEp) for the differential (Dacie and Lewis; NCCLS). The 95% confidence intervals for count and differential may be estimated from the following formulae:

$$\text{Poisson distribution} = \pm 1.84 \sqrt{n}$$

where 1.84 is a constant and N = number of cells counted

$$\text{SEp} = \pm 1.96 \sqrt{(p \times q)/n}$$

where 1.96 is a constant, p = proportion (percentage) of cells differentiated, q = 100 − p, and N = number of cells counted.

These simple relationships are fundamental to understanding the precision and accuracy provided by an automated hematology analyzer. In both counting and differentiating cells, the more cells counted, the more precise the result (Tables 7.1 and 7.2).

All automated leukocyte counting and differentiation can be traced to one of two lineages or can be a hybrid of both. These are bulk-flow aperture impedance (Coulter), focused flow light scatter (Crossland-Taylor), or combinations of both. Crossland-Taylor originally used a tungsten lamp with dark field illumination. Today, based on the work of van Dilla et al. (1969), the illumination is generally provided by a laser.

Table 7.1
Poisson Distribution

n	$\pm 1.84 \sqrt{n}$
10	±6
100	±18
1000	±58
10,000	±184
20,000	±260

Where n = number of events counted.

Counting and differentiating leukocytes in an automated hematology analyzer requires elimination of the predominant red blood cell (RBC) population (1000:1) plus detection and recognition of unique leukocyte characteristics. RBCs are typically eliminated by chemical and physical lysis or rendered optically transparent by hypotonic ghosting. The unique leukocyte characteristics can be native to the cell, amplified, or created by a chemical reaction.

At one time, the automated hematology analyzer provided a precise white blood cell (WBC) count, with the differential remaining an accurate yet less precise manual test. Those days are long gone, as all modern automated hematology analyzers generally include some differentiation of the leukocytes. This leukocyte differentiation may range from as few as two parts to as many as nine parts; each part being more or less accurate depending on the technology employed. Today, the clinician is typically provided with results from an indeterminate mix of precise automated and less precise manual, yet hopefully, accurate methods dictated by the interaction of the specimen, instrument and laboratory review criteria (Groner and Simson). With more complete and accurate automated differential analysis, there will be a concomitant decrease in the manual microscope component.

Table 7.2
Standard Error of Proportion SEp ± 1.96 $\sqrt{(pxq)/n}$

n	p	2	5	10	20
10		±9	±14	±19	±25
100		±3	±4	±6	±8
200		±2	±3	±4	±6
400		±1	±2	±3	±4
1000		±1	±1	±2	±2
5000		—	±1	±1	±1
10,000		—	—	±1	±1
20,000		—	—	—	±1

Where p = proportion (percentage) counted, q = 100 − p and n = number of events counted.

BULK FLOW APERTURE IMPEDANCE

Bulk flow direct current aperture impedance was first described by Coulter in 1956 and is now in use in numerous automated hematology analyzers manufactured by many companies throughout the world. In some analyzers, direct current impedance for measuring cytoplasmic volume has been combined with a radio-frequency signal to measure nuclear volume.

Following lysis of the more numerous red blood cells, the lysate modified leukocytes, suspended in an electrolyte, are pulled by a vacuum through a microscopic aperture between two electrodes. As leukocytes traverse the aperture, they momentarily impede direct current passing between the electrodes producing a detectable change in voltage (Fig. 7.1). The number of events is proportional to the leukocyte count and the change in voltage is essentially proportional to the volume of the leukocyte. Leukocytes taking a nonaxial passage through the aperture are oversized and create atypical pulses. These atypical pulses are discarded in an editing step. Recirculating leukocytes can be counted a second time as smaller cells. To prevent this occurrence, a second aperture is used to block the recirculation (von Behrens). The analog voltage pulses are converted into digital data by an analog to digital converter (ADC). To ensure that only the desired events are counted, excluding background electrical noise, stroma, or debris from lysis, the digitized data is compared to an internal standard and only those events above

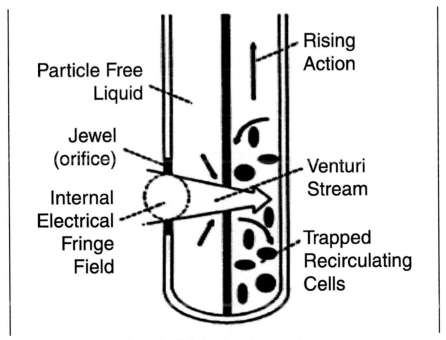

Figure 7.1. Bulk flow impedance aperture.

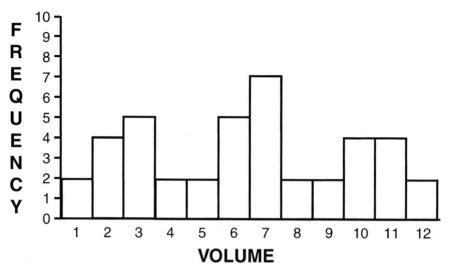

Figure 7.2. Volume frequency distribution—histogram.

a given "threshold voltage" are counted or further processed. The digitized data can be sorted by volume in a pulse height analyzer (Channelyzer) to yield a volume frequency distribution histogram (Fig. 7.2) depicting the after-lysis leukocyte volume distribution characteristics. The volume frequency distribution histogram can also be used to differentiate leukocytes by volume. Generating a leukocyte count requires that a recognized volume of known dilution be pulled through the aperture by a volumetric manometer and that the calculated concentration be corrected for any coincident passage. Coincidence occurs when more than one leukocyte occupies the aperture at the same time.

The degree of leukocyte differentiation that can be achieved by bulk flow aperture impedance is a function of the choice of lytic system (Table 7.3) and the sophistication of the algorithm employed to interrogate the result-

Table 7.3
Lysing Agents

Plant extract	Saponin
Organic acids	Formic acid, acetic acid
Quartenary ammonium salts	Ammonium chloride, ammonium oxalate, cetyltrimethylammonium bromide (Cetrimide)
Detergents & surfactants	Ionic, non-ionic, and mixed
Accelerators	Heat and hypotonicity
Retardants	Sodium bicarbonate
Fixatives	Formaldehyde, organic alcohols
Proprietary	Numerous patented formulations

ing leukocyte volume frequency distribution. In general, the more powerful the lytic reagent, the fewer the leukocyte populations that can be detected.

In the case of the Abbott Cell-Dyn 3500 system, a powerful lytic agent is used to eliminate any RBC or small platelet clumps that might resist a weaker lyse. This very powerful lyse strips cytoplasm from cells, leaving bare nuclei. The algorithm is designed to count all the nuclei, including all nucleated red blood cells (NRBCs), present in a single unimodal distribution (Fig. 7.3). The resulting total nucleated count, called WIC (WBC impedance count), can be used in conjunction with the Cell-Dyn 3500's gated optical WBC count, called WOC (WBC optical count) to flag and indirectly estimate NRBC (WIC greater than WOC flag NRBC; NRBC estimate WIC − WOC/WOC × 100).

Differentiation of leukocytes by direct current impedance measurement after physical separation from red cells was first described by van Dilla et al. (1967). Later, England et al. demonstrated lysis as an alternative to physical separation from red cells. Automated bimodal leukocyte volume distribution analysis was described as an "abridged" differential by Wycherly and O'Shea. They utilized the automated processing capabilities of the Coulter Model S and the analytic capabilities of the C-1000 Channelyzer to add rapid differentiation of lymphoid from myeloid cells to the then routine seven parameter complete blood (cell) count (CBC).

Today, the Cell-Dyn 1400 system uses a slightly attenuated lyse to create a bimodal direct current leukocyte volume distribution (Fig. 7.4). The first peak from the left in this distribution is lymphocytes and the second is the myeloid cells "granulocytes." Dividing the area under the first peak by the area under the entire distribution yields the percentage of lymphocytes. Dividing the area under the second peak by the entire area under the distribu-

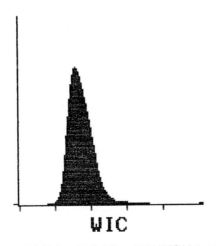

Figure 7.3. Unimodal Cell-Dyn 3500 WIC histogram.

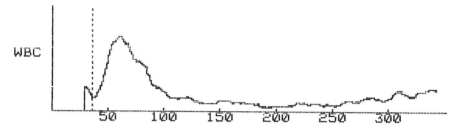

Figure 7.4. Bimodal Cell-Dyn 1400 histogram.

tion curve yields the percentage of granulocytes. The validity of the lymphocyte differentiation is verified by a "flagging" system. The "flagging" system checks for valleys on each side of the lymphocyte peak and to the left of the granulocyte peak and makes sure that these valleys are adequate, by comparing the counts in the peak with those in the valley (peak/valley ratio). Invalid lymphocyte or granulocyte separation generating a "flag" was seen as a potential indication of pathology and used as a trigger for manual smear review. Careful review of bimodal leukocyte distributions allowed astute observers to recognize the presence of blast cells in acute leukemia. Blast cells typically form a unique population, obscuring the normal valley between the lymphoid and myeloid cells. It was also possible to distinguish chronic lymphocytic leukemia (absolute lymphocytosis) from chronic granulocytic leukemia (absolute granulocytosis).

Further attenuation of the lytic reagent results in a tri-modal leukocyte direct current impedance volume distribution (Fig. 7.5). The tri-modal distribution, as seen in the Cell-Dyn 1700 system, is a result of partial lysis of the cell membrane, loss of cytoplasmic contents and shrinkage of the residual membrane around the nucleus and any granules that may be present. This technology is usually described as a "three-part diff." Attenuation of the lytic reagent also increases the potential for including un-lysed red cells and platelet clumps and some, but not necessarily all, of the NRBC in the count

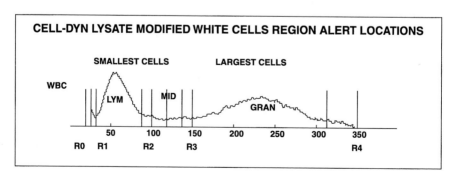

Figure 7.5. Trimodal Cell-Dyn 1700 histogram.

Table 7.4
Cell-Dyn 1700 flags

LYM RO: the region to the left of the expected valley below the lymphocyte peak
LYM R1: the region to the right of the expected valley below the lymphocyte peak
LYM R2: the region to the left of the expected valley above the lymphocyte peak
LYM RM: any combination of the above
MID R2: the region to the right of the expected valley above the lymphocyte peak
MID R3: the region to the left of the expected valley below the granulocyte peak
MID RM: any combination of the above
GRAN R3: the region to the right of the expected valley below the granulocyte peak
GRAN R4: the region to the left of the expected valley above the granulocyte peak
GRAN RM: any combination of the above

and differential (Cornbleet and Kessinger). The trimodal distribution results from expansion of the valley between lymphocytes and granulocytes into a third peak (wide plateau). This peak, the midsize cells, includes monocytes, eosinophils, basophils, blasts, and other precursors. The additional peak also creates another opportunity to test for adequate separation of the leukocyte subpopulations. With the Cell-Dyn 1700, the algorithm includes a check on each side of the expected valley positions and provides a series of flags, indicating any abnormality in the tri-modal volume distribution (Table 7.4). These flags for incomplete separation, due to subpopulation increases, decreases, spreads, and shifts, have been associated with pathology (Table 7.5).

Sasche and Henkel have characterized the Cell-Dyn 1700 as capable of detecting neutropenia related to myelosuppression and flagging the vast majority of samples with 3% or more of immature granulocytes, atypical lymphocytes, blasts, or NRBC (Sasche and Henkel).

Because of the association between flags and pathology, some manufacturers "translate" their instrument three-part leukocyte population distribu-

Table 7.5
Pathology Associated With Cell-Dyn 1700 flags

LYM RO may be caused by unlysed RBC, nucleated RBC, platelet clumps, giant platelets, cryoglobulins, or chronic lymphocytic leukemia
LYM R1 may be caused by lymphocytosis, lymphopenia, and cryoglobulins
LYM R2 may be caused by lymphocytosis, lymphopenia, blasts, plasma cells, variant lymphocytes, or basophilia
LYM RM: any combination of the above
MID R2 may be caused by lymphocytosis, lymphopenia, blasts, plasma cells, variant lymphocytes, basophilia, or monocytosis
MID R3 may be caused by eosinophilia, blasts, plasma cells, agranular neutrophils, basophilia, bands, or (occasionally) platelet clumps
MID RM: any combination of the above
GRAN R3 may be caused by granulocytosis, neutropenia, immature granulocytes, bands, eosinophilia, or agranular neutrophils
GRAN R4 may be caused by hypersegmented neutrophils, granulocytosis, or neutropenia
GRAN RM: any combination of the above

tion flags into more familiar morphologic terms, creating an "interpretive" differential. There is, however, no methodological improvement over a three-part differential reported as such. Furthermore, the interpretive differential can create a false sense of security by making the leukocyte differential seem more comprehensive than the data really allows.

In some systems, impedance to an alternating current at radio-frequency is added to measure nuclear volume simultaneously with direct current impedance measurement of cytoplasmic volume. The dual-parameter correlated data is then converted into an isometric histogram for three-part differential analysis. Additional aliquots of blood are subjected to changes in pH and the action of selected detergents creating bimodal direct current impedance volume distributions of others/eosinophils, others/basophils, and others/"immatures." The neutrophil percentage is calculated from granulocyte% less (eosinophil% plus basophil%). Flagging is generated from all four channels: three-part differential, eosinophils, basophils, and immatures (Sysmex).

While the use of the "three-part diff" is declining in larger institutions that have upgraded to the automated five-part differential, its use is increasing in primary care. This is because evermore cost-effective three-part differential systems are being developed (Cell-Dyn 1200 system). Since primary care givers see patients on presentation, the first referral of suspected acute leukemia is likely to include the results from a three-part differential system. Wherever possible, in addition to noting the almost inevitable neutropenia and increase in midsize cells, review of this data should include the leukocyte volume distribution histogram and flags. This is important baseline information as the tri-modal histogram is analogous to the orthogonal (90°) light scatter data generated by a flow cytometer and some five-part automated differential analyzers (Fig. 7.6). Orthogonal (90°) light scatter is similar to the attenuated lyse volume distribution in that both recognize differences in the lobularity of the nucleus and granularity of the cytoplasm.

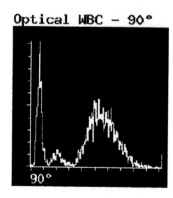

Figure 7.6. Trimodal Cell-Dyn 4000 90° light scatter histogram.

Thus, comparison of volume distribution and light scatter data provides a valuable link between primary and tertiary care. Furthermore, the skill acquired in the review of trimodal leukocyte volume distribution histograms is transferable to the interpretation of light scatter data.

FOCUSED FLOW LIGHT SCATTER AND FLUORESCENCE

The dark-field, or light scatter, technique of microscopy was once common in clinical laboratory use for the detection of spirochetes and trypanosomes. In dark-field microscopy, a beam stop prevents light from a tungsten-lamp from passing through the parasite to the objective. Thus, the objective collects only the light scattered so that in the eyepiece, a bright parasite may be seen against a dark background. Leukocytes in a wet preparation are seen exceptionally well by this method, because their granules are refractile and set off the nucleus in sharp contrast (Hansen-Prus).

Fluorescence microscopy is also a dark-field technique. Optical filters are used to restrict the incident light from a mercury arc lamp to the short wavelengths needed for excitation and allow only the longer wavelengths resulting from emission to reach the eyepiece. While autofluorescence may be studied, it is more usual to stain cells for properties of interest. In the clinical laboratory, Auromine O has been used to look for acid fast bacilli and fluorescein isothiocyanate labeled antihuman globulin used to look for autoantibodies to tissues.

Many attempts were made to create a cell counter by combining an electrical photodetector, dark-field microscopy and the passage of cells through a capillary. These attempts were largely unsuccessful, due to coincident passage of cells in a large bore capillary and frequent sample blockage in a small bore capillary. Crossland-Taylor solved these problems with the introduction of hydrodynamic focusing.

In hydrodynamic focusing, a suspension of cells is slowly injected into a faster moving stream of fluid moving in the same direction. As a result of laminar flow, the cell suspension does not mix with the surrounding "sheath." As the flow of the faster moving sheath stream is constricted, it accelerates the slower moving cells and focuses them into a coaxial, yet single, file as they pass an observation point (Fig. 7.7). Thus, focused flow solves the problems of coincidence and nonaxial passage inherent in both optical and impedance counting.

Interest in the measurement of cellular DNA content for rapid detection of malignancy led van Dilla to combine the focused flow cell with fluorescent measurement of DNA content. A short wavelength argon laser was used to excite a fluorescent DNA stain and a sensitive photomultiplier was used to detect the emission from both Chinese hamster ovary cells and normal human leukocytes. The flow cell was perpendicular to the horizontal laser beam. Measurement of fluorescence was made in the same horizontal plane, but at right angles, that is, orthogonal to the laser beam. The use of

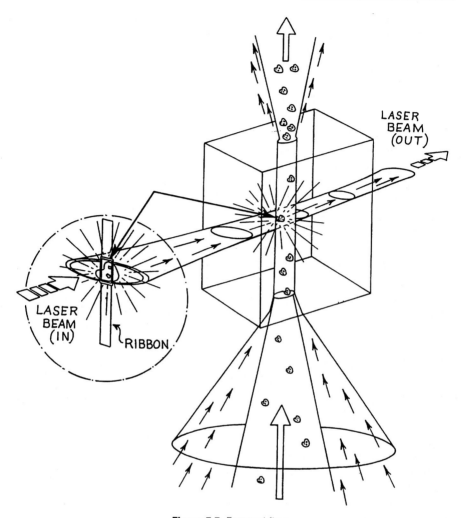

Figure 7.7. Focused flow.

a laser, which has a coherent (nondivergent) and stable light output over long periods of time, also solved the older problems of focusing a mercury lamp on a small observation point and diminishing lamp intensity over time. Measurement of cell volume was made on a separate aliquot of sample by using direct current impedance. The frequency distributions of nuclear fluorescence and cytoplasmic volume were overlaid for comparison. In 1968, these authors anticipated the extension of the method to include multiparameter analysis by combination with small-angle light scatter. More recently (1996), red fluorescence from propidium iodide, axial light loss and 7° scatter have been used to count NRBC and determine leukocyte viability in an automated hematology analyzer (Kim et al.).

With use of the laser established by van Dilla, others went on to show that near forward angle light scattering could be used to measure cell size (Mullaney et al.) and that a combination of forward and orthogonal scatter could be used to differentiate leukocytes into lymphocytes, monocytes, and granulocytes (Salzman et al.). Later, it was shown that rotation of the plane of polarized light could be used to differentiate granulocytes into neutrophils and eosinophils (Terstappen et al.). Similar three or four-part differentiation has been accomplished using: impedance and radio-frequency, impedance and scatter, and peroxidase activity and scatter. Peroxidase activity is measured by absorbance combined with tungsten light scatter (Mansberg et al.). Here the cost of the test is moved from the instrument hardware to the reagent system.

Laser is an acronym for light amplification by stimulated emission radiation. Lasers come in many sizes, types, and price ranges. The two lasers most commonly used in the clinical laboratory are the helium-neon (HeNe) and argon ion. The HeNe laser emits red light at 633 nm and is used in applications where only light scatter is to be measured. It is relatively inexpensive and does not need a large power supply. In contrast, the more expensive argon ion laser which requires a large power supply emits blue light at 488 nm and is used in applications when fluorescence is to be measured in addition to scatter. Light scattered at near forward angles can be detected with inexpensive photodiode(s). Right angle or orthogonal light scatter and fluorescence require a more expensive photomultiplier with its associated power supply for detection. These differences lead to the differences in the cost of automated hematology analyzers. Bulk flow aperture impedance is relatively inexpensive, needing only the aperture and a pair of electrodes. Focusing the flow increases cost somewhat and adding forward angle light scatter with straight through photo diode detectors increases it a little more. Addition of orthogonal scatter requires a sophisticated optical bench to hold the components in spatial alignment, plus the addition of photomultiplier(s) and their associated power supply, increasing cost still more. Ultimately, and at maximum cost, measurement of fluorescence requires argon laser excitation and additional photomultiplier(s) to measure the fluorescent emission. In 1988, Shapiro estimated that it would take approximately 2 months and cost around $25,000 to home-build an argon ion laser based flow cytometer (20). This, of course, requires adjustment for inflation and does not include all the additional components required to automate a CBC!

The flashes of scattered and fluorescent light produced at the flow cell are converted into voltage pulses by the photodetector(s) and their associated amplifiers. These amplifiers are typically linear for light scatter and always logarithmic for fluorescence. This is because variation of light scatter remains linear within an order of magnitude (myeloid cells are twice the volume of lymphoid cells); whereas, fluorescence is logarithmic spanning many orders of magnitude (non-viable leukocytes and NRBCs are 10 to 100 times brighter than unstained cells). The analog signals representing the cells must cross a single voltage or multiple voltage thresholds for acceptance and subsequent conversion into digital format by an A/D converter (ADC). The digital format is used for all further analysis and storage. This process of digitizing the analog data is often referred to as "channelyzing the data," although "channelyzing" is also used to mean displaying the data as a population frequency distribution histogram.

Single parameter data, as exemplified by bulk flow impedance, is conveniently analyzed and displayed as a frequency distribution histogram. This is typically the number of events in each channel over a range of 256 channels. Storing this data for later review requires 256 numbers or bits of information, considerably less than the result for each of the thousands of cells originally analyzed. In such a population frequency distribution, each cell has lost its individual identity and is analyzed as part of a one-dimensional population. This is all very well for single parameter data, however, the essence of flow cytometry is to collect more than one parameter simultaneously.

With two parameters, data can be stored as dual parameter correlated data, that is two population frequency distributions that may be analyzed and displayed in a matrix (Table 7.6). Since dual parameter correlated data is often used when processing power and storage are limited, the data is often reduced still further to a 64 × 64 matrix. Again, each cell has lost its individual identity and is being analyzed as part of a two-dimensional population. Any box in the matrix shows the sum of cells with both characteristics, it cannot show which individuals had each characteristic or to what extent.

Table 7.6
Matrix From Dual Parameter Correlated Data

Single Parameter Data												
Channel	1	2	3	4	5	6	7	8	9	10	11	12
y	2	4	5	2	2	5	7	2	2	4	4	2
x	2	8	9	2	2	10	12	2	1	3	3	1

Bold lines are valleys between populations in single parameter data.

Dual Parameter Matrix												
12	4	9	11	4	4	12	14	4	3	5	5	3
11	6	12	13	6	6	14	16	6	5	7	7	5
10	6	12	13	6	6	14	16	6	5	7	7	5
9	4	9	11	4	4	12	14	4	3	5	5	3
8	4	9	11	4	4	12	14	4	3	5	5	3
7	9	12	16	9	9	17	19	9	8	10	10	8
6	9	13	14	7	7	15[a]	17	7	6	8	8	6
5	4	10	11	4	4	12	14	4	3	5	5	3
4	4	10	11	4	4	12	14	4	3	5	5	3
3	7	13	14	7	7	15	17	7	6	8	8	6
2	6	12	13	6	6	14	16	6	5	7	7	5
1	4	10	11	4	4	12	14	4	3	5	5	3
Channel	1	2	3	4	5	6	7	8	9	10	11	12

[a] Sum of x channel 6 and y channel 6, 10 + 5 = 15.
Bold lines are intersecting projections of valleys from single parameter data.

Table 7.7
List Mode Data

Cell	0° Size	10° N/C Ratio	90° Lobularity	90°D Granularity	Log FL3 Red Fluorescence
1	165	162	150	30	30
2	60	65	15	5	64
3	140	80	30	7	92
4	150	180	125	110	100
5	100	110	35	5	46
6	36	37	8	4	212

So, given that there might be four or five measured parameters for each cell, how can this data best be handled? Recording multiple parameters on thousands of cells is best accomplished using a list mode format. Each cell is identified by number and each characteristic is recorded individually, forming a table or "list" (Table 7.7). In this way, each cell is identified by its own unique characteristics and not lost in a population of its fellows.

List mode data is typically displayed as an x-y scatterplot, with each dot

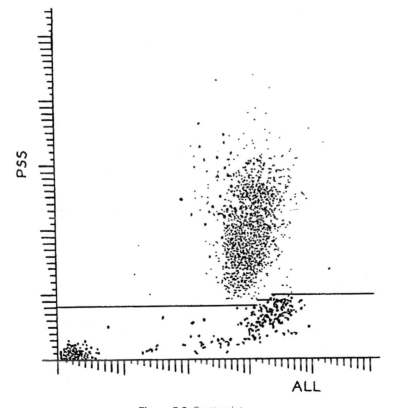

Figure 7.8. Scatterplot.

representing the location of a single cell (Fig. 7.8). With increasing concentration of a single cell type the location on the scatterplot can become very dense and "burn-out." For this reason, contour plots, similar to elevation maps, are sometimes used for display (Fig. 7.9). Since list mode data is correlated data and one parameter can be compared to others, it is possible to answer questions such as how many agranular cells are large and low in lobularity (blasts) or how many mononuclear cells are small and highly fluorescent (NRBC).

The use of correlated data where multiple parameters are measured on a single cell can be contrasted to the use of collated data. Collated data results from the use of multiple channels to make multiple measurements on multiple aliquots of sample. This population data is then used to calculate a final differential result. Some instruments in use today use collated data from multiple channels to calculate a final leukocyte differential (Table 7.8).

Generating a leukocyte differential from scatterplot and list mode data is accomplished by the process of gating. The scatterplots may be gated in single or multiple steps. These steps typically follow in sequence and the out-

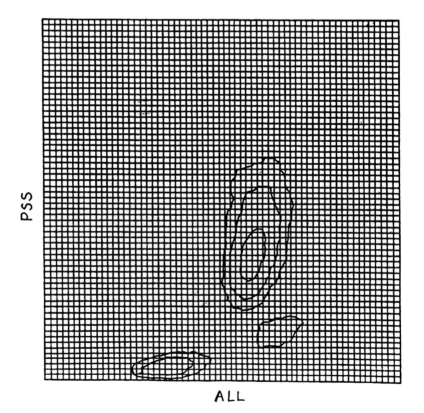

Figure 7.9. Contour plot.

Table 7.8
Collated Data Systems

Manufacturer	Channels
Sysmex SE-9000	Impedance WBC Lym/mono/gran EO BASO Immatures
Technicon H*Series	Peroxidase Basophil/lobularity

come at each step is recorded in list mode. This process is described as sequential multiparameter analysis.

The most simple gates are straight lines drawn onto the scatterplot from projections of original single parameter data. These lines are frequently projected from the valleys between single parameter histograms. The intersection of these lines creates a rectangle or series of rectangles creating a tic-tac-toe or noughts-and-crosses appearance. All cells within a given rectangle or rectangles are then assigned to a designated classification and this classification is noted in the list mode table. The classification may be preliminary or final. If preliminary, the cells selected may be re-projected in a further scatterplot of additional parameters, allowing a further classification and notation in list mode. This sequential process of gating and re-projection continues until all the cells are classified and/or all the parameter combinations are exhausted.

There are many alternatives to rectangular gating; these include: isometric gates, radial gates, distance gates, circles, quadrants, ellipses, and bit-mapping (Fig. 7.10a–e). Isometric gates are created by projecting the scatterplot data onto any new plane to form an entirely new histogram. Radial gates may be drawn using the angle of each cell from a predetermined origin, creating a pie slice across the scatterplot. Distance from the origin within the radial slice creates a defined segment. Circles, quadrants, and ellipses can be constructed at given distances, often determined by population statistics, from the actual or expected mode of a population. In bit-mapping, the scatterplot is converted into a contour plot and a zig-zag line is drawn around the lowest contour between populations. These methods of gating may be used alone or in combination, depending on the complexity of the scatterplots to be analyzed.

Sequential multi-variate analysis is a one way process from start to finish; however, in leukocyte differentiation, it is often necessary to change, or validate, an earlier classification made in one dimension based on the result of a later step in another dimension. Changing classifications in process is known as systematic multivariate analysis.

For ease of visual interpretation, cells in list mode are six color coded (five

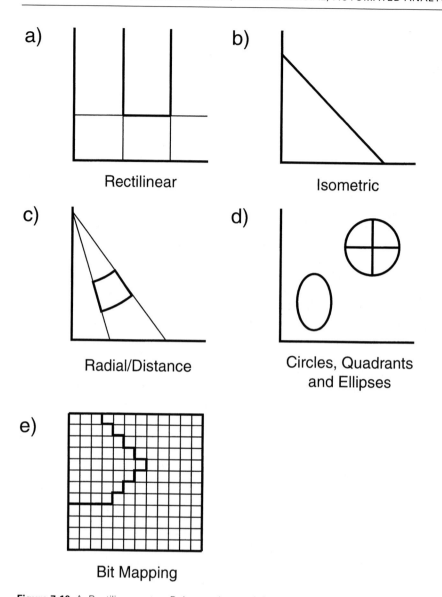

Figure 7.10. A. Rectilinear gates. B. Isometric gates. C. Radial/distance gates. D. Circles, quadrants, and ellipses. E. Bit mapping.

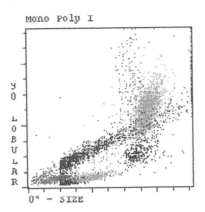

Figure 7.11. Color scatterplot.

normal leukocytes, non-white blood cells and NRBC) and are projected as final scatterplots (Fig. 7.11). This allows an observer to see the results of multivariate analysis, that is, mixed and overlapping margins between different colored cell types in simple two-dimensional color scatterplots. Dual parameter correlated data is sometimes color coded; however, this results in population-specific rather than cell-specific color. With dual parameter correlated data, mixed and overlapping margins between different colored cell types are never seen.

The additional populations revealed by multi-parameter data create additional opportunities to test for adequate separation, increased heterogeneity, or additional leukocyte subpopulations. Finding inadequate separation of subpopulations due to shifts, spreads, or additions usually results from the presence of immature cells and generates a "morphology" flag. Some instruments, however, inhibit reporting the affected leukocyte subpopulation, whereas others inhibit the entire differential.

Immature leukocytes, especially blasts, are generally larger than more mature cells. If present in small numbers, immature cells increase the heterogeneity of a subpopulation with respect to size and, if present in sufficient numbers, increase the average size of that subpopulation. In this regard, detecting immature leukocytes is analogous to the early detection of abnormal RBC morphology with changes in red blood cell distribution width (RDW) preceding changes in mean cell volume (MCV) (Bessman et al.). Much morphological flagging is, therefore, based on size distribution and average size data (Table 7.9).

The success of morphological flagging is dependent on the quality of the initial separation into neutrophils, lymphocytes, monocytes, eosinophils, and basophils. Successful detection of blasts requires recognition as a mononuclear cell, rather than a granulocyte, followed by recognition of an abnormal size distribution or other parameters indicative of blasts. Other charac-

Table 7.9
Generalized Morphological Flagging Based on Size

Morphological Flag	Description Based on Size	Parameters
NRBC	Smaller than lymphocytes after lysis	Increase in percentage or number at or below a gate
Bands	Larger neutrophils	Moderate increase in mean Moderate increase in S.D.* Increase in percentage or number at or above a gate
Immature granulocytes	Very large neutrophils	Marked increase in mean Marked increase in S.D. Increase in percentage or number at or above a higher gate
Variant lymphocytes	Large lymphocytes	Moderate increase in mean Moderate increase in S.D.
Blasts	Very large monocytes	Marked increase in mean Marked increase in S.D. Increase in percentage or number at or above a gate

*S.D. = standard deviation.

teristics that may be used to flag abnormal mononuclear cells as blasts include the percentage mononuclears, the number of mononuclears, the heterogeneity of nuclear to cytoplasmic ratio, the heterogeneity of lobularity, and the degree of membrane permeability.

Discriminant functions using light scatter and fluorescence data can be used to flag blasts and other immature cells. Since discriminant functions generate a numerical result, they may be used to report a normalized confidence fraction in addition to the morphological flag. Discriminant functions, using CBC data, have long been used to distinguish iron deficiency from beta thalassemia trait (Table 7.10).

Depending on the sensitivity and specificity of the flag and the population being tested, manual microscopy may be required for confirmation or for when enumeration of immature cells is required. Enumeration of blasts and other immature cells is almost always required for the detection, diagnosis,

Table 7.10
Discriminant Functions

	Thalassemia Trait	Iron Deficiency
Mentzer Index: MCV/RBC	<13	>13
Shine and Lal: $(MCV)^2 \times MCH$	<1530	>1530
England and Fraser: $MCV - RBC - (5 \times Hgb) - 8.4$	Negative values	Positive values

Table 7.11
Cell-Dyn 3000 Series Systems Comparison

	Cell-Dyn 3000	Cell-Dyn 3500	Cell-Dyn 3200
Open sample volume	170 μL	130 μL	120 μL
Closed sample volume	230 μL	240 μL	250 μL
Optional loader			
sample volume	350 μL	355 μL	250 μL
capacity	100 samples	100 samples	50 samples
Maximum thruput	72/hour	90/hour	70/hour
WBC	WOC	WIC & WOC	WOC (reflex [a]NOC)
Differential	[b]M.A.P.S.S.	M.A.P.S.S.	M.A.P.S.S.
RBC/PLT	Impedance	Impedance	Optical
Reticulocytes	No	Yes	Planned

[a] NOC, nucleated optical count.
[b] M.A.P.S.S., Multi-angle Polarized Scatter Separation.

and treatment of acute leukemia. Such enumeration of blasts and other immature cells as part of a routine leukocyte count and differential is now technically feasible. The methodologies used are instrument specific and are described in the next section.

Cell-Dyn 3000 series

The Cell-Dyn 3000 series of automated hematology analyzers comprises three different, yet similar systems: the original Cell-Dyn 3000; the later Cell-Dyn 3500; and, most recently, the Cell-Dyn 3200 (Fig. 7.12a–c; Table 7.11).

All Cell-Dyn 3000 series systems utilize the same leukocyte reagent system, flow cell, helium-neon laser, and optical bench (Fig. 7.13).

Dilution in a hypotonic salt solution (SHEATH REAGENT) is used to dehemoglobinize red cells, rendering them invisible to laser light (where hypotonically resistant red cells are present [neonates; sickle cells], an operator selectable Resistant Red Blood Cell mode extends incubation time [Joyner and Brooks; Dorner et al.]). A syringe metered volume of the resulting cell suspension, doubled to increase precision if the WBC is less than 2.0×10^9/L, is injected through the flow cell.

Light scatter exceeding a 0° hardware threshold is detected, digitized, counted as raw events, and also used to determine count rate. Increasing count rate indicates obstruction of the flow cell, decreasing count rate indicates the presence of hypotonically sensitive "fragile" leukocytes. Light scatter at all four angles 0°, 10°, 90°, and 90° depolarized is detected, digitized, and recorded in list mode format for up to 10,000 events (Fig. 7.14a–c).

Sequential list mode analysis (Fig. 7.12A–C) differentiates cells into

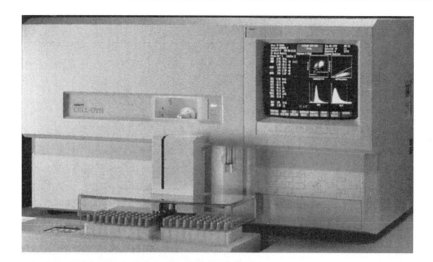

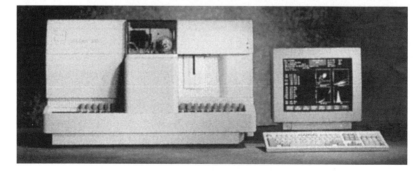

Figure 7.12. A. Cell-Dyn 3000. B. Cell-Dyn 3500. C. Cell-Dyn 3200.

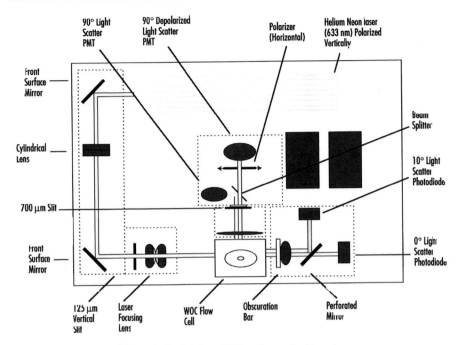

Figure 7.13. Cell-Dyn 3000 series optical bench.

mononuclears (agranular cells) and polymorphonuclears (granular cells) by an isometric histogram of 90° (lobularity) and 10° (nuclear to cytoplasmic ratio) light scatter. Polymorphonuclears (granular cells) are differentiated into eosinophils and neutrophils by radial analysis of 90° depolarized (granularity) and 90° (lobularity) light scatter. The mononuclears (agranular cells) are further differentiated into lymphocytes, monocytes, intentionally degranulated basophils, and nonleukocytes (NWBC) by a rectilinear and isometric analysis of 0° (size) and 10° (nuclear to cytoplasmic ratio) light scatter. Any nonleukocytes, NRBC, giant platelets, platelet clumps, or residual hypotonically resistant RBC, are gated out of the leukocyte count and differential.

Blasts (large mononuclear cells) are estimated using a predefined region of the 90° (lobularity) and 0° (size) scatterplot. A blast region estimate greater than 1.0% or monocytes greater than 20.0% trigger a morphological flag.

Immature granulocytes and bands (large polymorphonuclear cells) are estimated using quadrants constructed around the neutrophil population in 0° (size) and 10° (nuclear to cytoplasmic ratio) scatter. An immature granulocyte region estimate greater than 3.0%, band region estimate greater than 12.5%, or greater than 50% of the neutrophils trigger a morphological flag.

Variant lymphocytes are estimated using the difference between the measured and expected lymphocyte 0° (size) distributions or the difference between the kinetic-corrected leukocyte count (due to a declining count rate) and the measured leukocyte count. A variant lymphocyte estimate greater

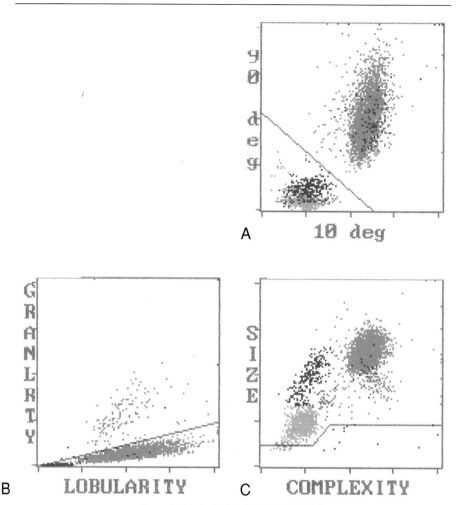

Figure 7.14. A. 90/10. B. 90/90. C. 0/10.

than 10.0% triggers a morphological flag.

Immature cell region estimates are for laboratory use and displayed on a Flagging Diagnostics Screen (Fig. 7.15). Flagging Diagnostics Region Estimates have been shown to be reproducible in leukopenic patients (Jones et al.).

Cell-Dyn 4000®

The Cell-Dyn 4000® automated hematology analyzer (Fig. 7.16) differs from the Cell-Dyn 3000 series in the use of an argon-ion laser as the light source and the ability to measure red (FL3) and green (FL1) fluorescence. Axial light loss (AxLL, 0° light loss) is used instead of forward angle light scatter (FALS) to measure relative size (Fig. 7.17); however, due to space restrictions this is described as 0° size on the Cell-Dyn 4000® scatterplots. Seven de-

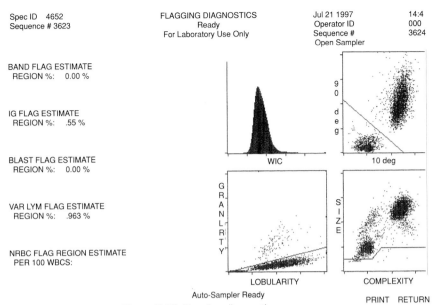

Figure 7.15. Flagging diagnostics screen.

gree light scatter is used instead of 10° scatter to measure nuclear to cytoplasmic ratio. Measurement of 90° and 90° depolarized scatter for lobularity and granularity, respectively, is similar (Fig. 7.18).

A novel leukocyte reagent system lyses the erythrocyte cytoplasmic membrane, stains any bare erythroblast nuclei or nonviable (permeable) leukocytes with propidium iodide, and fixes both the stained and unstained nu-

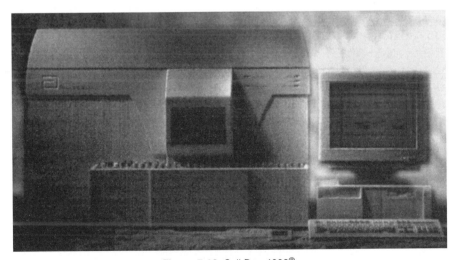

Figure 7.16. Cell-Dyn 4000®.

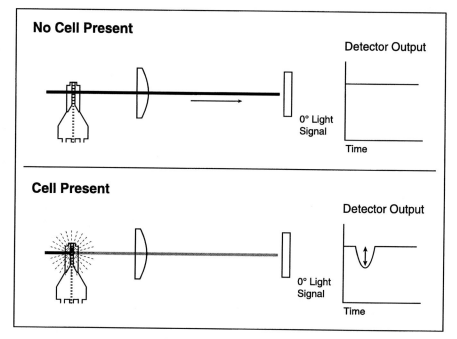

Figure 7.17. Axial light loss.

cleated cells prior to flow cytometric analysis. Propidium iodide is excluded from viable (nonpermeable) leukocytes by an intact cytoplasmic membrane. Propidium iodide bound to nuclear DNA generates red fluorescence (FL3) when excited with argon-laser light.

A syringe metered volume of the lysed and stained cell suspension is injected through the flow cell. (The operator may elect to quadruple this volume using the extended WBC count mode. This mode is intended for rare event analysis.) Stroma and debris from lysis are eliminated by a unique triple trigger threshold since only signals exceeding a 7° scatter threshold and 0° light loss or FL3 red fluorescence threshold circuit are digitized, used to determine raw count, count rate, and recorded in list mode format for up to 20,000 events.

Systematic list mode analysis (Fig. 7.19A–D) differentiates the cells into mononuclears (agranular cells) and polymorphonuclears (granular cells) primarily by a bit-mapping approach using 90° (lobularity) and 7° (nuclear to cytoplasmic ratio) light scatter. This decision is validated with 90° scatter/0° loss and 0° loss/7° scatter data.

The very small, highly fluorescent, bare erythroblast nuclei are excluded from the mononuclear fraction by a rectangular two-dimensional gate and, therefore, are not included in the leukocyte or differential counts. This decision is validated with proprietary multiparameter, multiweighted, discrim-

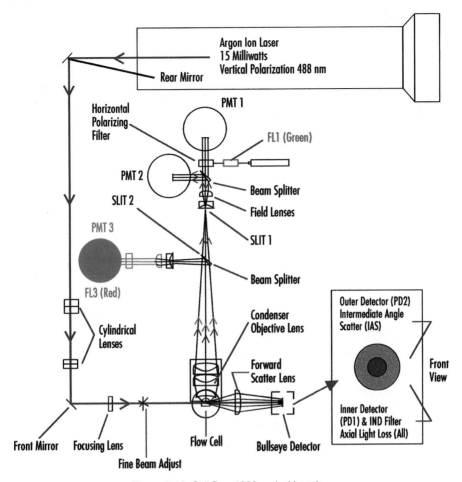

Figure 7.18. Cell-Dyn 4000 optical bench.

inant functions. The larger, less intensely staining, nonviable (permeable) leukocytes are included with the unstained viable (nonpermeable) leukocytes in the total leukocyte count and differential.

Polymorphonuclears (granular cells) are differentiated into neutrophils and eosinophils by radial analysis using 90° depolarized and 90° light scatter. This decision is also validated with 90° scatter/0° loss and 0° loss/7° scatter data.

The mononuclears (agranular cells) are differentiated into monocytes and non-leukocytes by finding an upper and lower valley in the single parameter histogram of 0° light loss. The remaining mononuclears are further differentiated into lymphocytes, basophils, and nonleukocytes by two-dimensional isometric analysis of 0° light loss and 7° light scatter plus radial analysis of 90° scatter and 0° light loss.

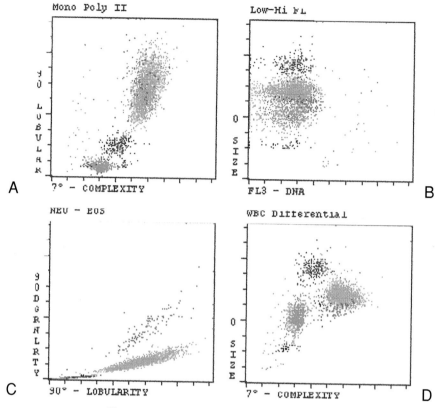

Figure 7.19. A. 90/7. B. 0/FL3. C. 90/90. D. 0/7.

Nonleukocytes, such as platelet clumps and/or lyse-resistant RBC, are gated from the leukocyte count and differential. (Samples with lyse resistant RBC may be run in a resistant RBC mode, which prolongs lysing time, chemically eliminating them from the count and differential.) Platelet clumps and lyse-resistant RBC generate specific flags (pltCLMP and rstRBC). Any other particle, such as bone marrow fat, not meeting identifiable multidimensional criteria is ruled "out of bounds." Particles ruled "out of bounds" generate an invalid data flag and are excluded from the leukocyte count and differential.

The viable leukocyte fraction (WBC viable fraction), is determined from the ratio of unstained to total leukocytes. If the WVF is less than 90%, a nonviable flag is generated.

Blasts, immature granulocytes, bands, and variant lymphocytes are detected by a proprietary multiparameter, multiweighted discriminant function that generates a flag and reports a confidence fraction from 0.50 to 0.99. Following detection by the discriminant function, blasts (large mononuclear cells) are primarily estimated by using 90° scatter and 0° light loss. The immature granulocytes and bands (large polymorphonuclear cells) are primarily estimated by using 0° loss and 7° light scatter. The variant lymphocytes (heterogeneous and/or permeable) are primarily estimated using 0° light loss and red fluorescence (FL3). Performance characteristics for the Cell-Dyn 4000® blast and variant lymphocyte flags are provided in the operations manual (Table 7.12A–E).

In spiking experiments, when cultured leukemic blasts cells were added to an otherwise normal peripheral blood sample, the Cell-Dyn 4000® was able to recover 3.6%, or 0.1×10^9/L (Glazier et al.). Furthermore, even at a concentration of 0.8% or 0.025×10^9/L, a few events easily distinguishable from the donor's monocytes could be seen in the blast region of the scatterplot. In this study, regression analysis showed good agreement between the Cell-Dyn 4000® blast region estimate and the expected value ($r^2 = 0.97$, slope = 0.98, intercept = -1.17).

D'Onofrio et al. have shown that the Cell-Dyn 4000® blast flag and confidence fraction (at 0.99) are sensitive and specific for bone marrow samples having more than 5% blasts (Table 7.13).

APPLICATION

Morphological flags with medically acceptable false-negative rates and economically acceptable false-positive rates, used in combination with other CBC data, are useful for screening. Utility for screening decreases, however, as the prevalence of abnormals in a population increases. In addition, flags, even if modified by confidence fractions, have only two states—ON and OFF. A false positive may result from exceeding a flag's trigger value by a fraction of a percent. Conversely, a false negative may result from missing the trigger value by a fraction of a percent. False positives can be reduced by inspection of the scatterplot, "interpretation" of the confidence fraction, and consideration of concurrent or comparison to previous CBC data. False negatives can be reduced by careful inspection of the scatterplot and consideration of concurrent or comparison to previous CBC data.

In screening for acute leukemia, it is customary for predetermined automated hematology analyzer review criteria to result in reflex slide examination by a medical technologist. The analyzer review criteria generally include any blood count and differential parameters outside of reference intervals, plus all morphological flags. Medical technologist microscopic confirmation of a medically significant new abnormality then results in hematopathology review.

The predetermined review criteria are generally set so that large numbers of slides are reviewed with the intention of minimizing any false negatives. In this expensive, time-consuming process, two sets of review criteria are in operation. These are the analyzer criteria for medical technologist slide review and the medical technologist's slide criteria for hematopathology re-

Table 7.12 A–E
Performance Characteristics—Blast and Var Lym Flags

A

Blast Flag Sensitivity

Reference Differential Result	N	CELL–DYN 4000® Sensitivity
≥1%	42	83.3%
≥5%	30	90.0%†
≥10%	24	91.7%†

† See following table.

B

Analysis of Blast Flag False Negatives ≥5% (from the previous table.)

Specimen ID	WBC		BLAST % Ref. Manual Differential	IG % Ref. Manual Differential	CELL-DYN 4000® VAR LYM Flag	CELL-DYN 4000® IG Flag
	S.I.	U.S.				
A19225	1.3×10^9/L	1.3×10^3/µL	22	0	Yes	No
A19953	6.1×10^9L	6.1×10^3/µL	9	23	No	Yes
A20035	2.4×10^9/L	2.4×10^3/µL	51	0	Yes	No

C

Variant Lymphocyte Flag Sensitivity

Reference Manual Differential	N	CELL–DYN 4000® Sensitivity
≥6%	41	48.8%
≥8%	23	69.6%
≥10%	20	80.0%
≥15%	12	91.7%

D

Variant Lymphocyte Flag Sensitivity (Using VAR LYM or Blast Flag)

Reference Manual Differential (% Variant Lymphocytes)	N	Cell-DYN 4000® Sensitivity
≥6%	41	63.4%
≥8%	23	73.9%
≥10%	20	80.0%
≥15%	12	91.7%

E

Specificity

Flag	N	Specificity
BAND	90	94.4%
IG	90	94.4%
BLAST	90	99.2%

Table 7.13
Efficiency of Blast Flag in Marrow

Morphology	Blast Flag Negative	Blast Flag Positive <0.99	Blast Flag Positive at 0.99	Total
Blasts <5%	45	18	1	64
Blasts >5%	0	7	13	20
Total	45	25	14	84

view. Much medical technologist microscopic review is a quality control check on the output of the analyzer. Medical technologist microscopic review will hopefully find anything the analyzer missed and, in rejecting any false positive result, will save needless hematopathology review. Such medical technologist review is expensive, tedious, tiring, and subject to statistical limitations in finding the infrequent cell types described earlier. With the sophisticated analysis provided by today's hematology analyzers, the need for medical technologist microscopic detection and confirmation of an abnormality prior to hematopathology review is questionable.

Today's hematology analyzers can be trusted to screen for acute leukemia because of their ability to accurately recognize and count the polymorphonuclear neutrophils while separating them from the mononuclear blasts. There should no longer be any concern that acute leukemia might be mistaken for a moderate reactive neutrophilia without medical technologist microscopic review. Neither should there be concern that platelet clumping will be reported as a pseudo-leukocytosis with a pseudo-thrombocytopenia since recent hematology analyzers gate platelet clumps from the WBC and flag for platelet clumps (Bowen et al.).

In patients presenting with neutropenia, anemia, and thrombocytopenia; with or without lymphocytosis and a variant lymphocyte flag; or monocytosis and a blast flag, hematopathology review is required. To eliminate unnecessary pathology reviews, medical technologists should be empowered to determine if pancytopenia is the result of chemotherapy, or if immature granulocyte and blast flags are the result of colony stimulating factor (CSF).

Acute promyelocytic leukemia FAB M3 should be suspected in patients presenting with neutrophilia, anemia, and thrombocytopenia where the laboratory report indicates that immature granulocytes are predominant and blasts are suspected with a high confidence fraction. Again, to eliminate unnecessary hematopathology review, chemotherapy and CSF may have to be excluded, as these often result in a blood count and scatterplot resembling acute promyelocytic or chronic myelogenous leukemia. Nevertheless, FAB M3 is invariably associated with coagulation abnormalities.

Medical technologists should be trained and encouraged to recognize the blood count and scatterplot appearances typical of acute and chronic leukemia. In 1974, Mansberg et al. observed that scatterplots were a valuable diagnostic aid to the blood count and that rules for their interpretation could be taught very quickly.

We have the opportunity to revise the two-step slide review process to a single step. We might replace the analyzer criteria for medical technologist review followed by the medical technologist criteria for hematopathology review with: blood count and scatterplot review criteria applied by medical technologists for microscopic hematopathology review.

The hematopathologist has a key role in determining the hematology analyzer blood count and scatterplot medical review criteria and in training the medical technologists to interpret automated blood count and scatterplot information.

FUTURES

The analysis of multidimensional light scatter information beyond a five-part differential has only begun in the last few years. The practical knowledge gained from having large numbers of laser light scatter systems in hematology laboratories throughout the world is immense. Large libraries of list mode data are now available for research and development. It is not unreasonable to expect laser light scatter methodologies to provide a reportable nine-part differential in the not too distant future (Fig. 7.20).

The inclusion of propidium iodide fluorescence in a routine hematology analyzer has already added a reportable NRBC count and laboratory indication of cell viability. It is likely that cell viability measurements will find a role in demonstrating the effectiveness of chemotherapy in acute leukemia.

With the measurement of fluorescence established on a hematology analyzer, any test performed on a flow cytometer is a candidate for transfer to the fluorescent hematology analyzer. It is, however, more likely that high volume routine tests and tests unique to the routine hematology service will be developed for the fluorescent hematology analyzer.

The high volume tests for persons infected with human immunodeficiency virus (HIV), include $CD3^+/CD4^+$ and $CD3^+/CD8^+$. Expanding the immunodeficiency panel with $CD3^-/CD19^+$ for B cells and $CD3^-/CD16^+$ or $CD3^-/CD56^+$ for NK cells (CDC) may have some utility for indicating the lineage of acute leukemia.

Unique tests for the hematology service include CD61 reference immunofluorescent platelet count (Ault et al.) and CD64 activated neutrophils (Davis et al.).

A CD45 reference immunofluorescent leukocyte count, with CD14 immunofluorescent monocytes is a good starting point for the reference immunofluorescent differential (Hubl et al.). The reference immunofluorescent differential would in turn provide a basis for distinguishing AML from ALL by the addition of further myeloid markers such as CD33; however, an immunofluorescent antibody to myeloperoxidase may be of more value than a panel of surface markers in rapidly distinguishing AML from ALL.

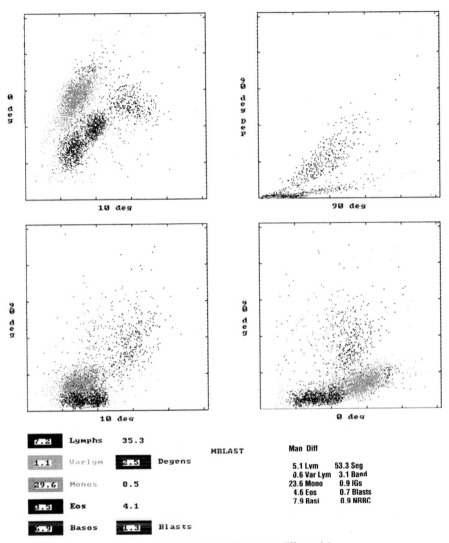

Figure 7.20. Nine-part light scatter differential.

BIBLIOGRAPHY

Ault KA, Mitchell J, Knowles C, et al. Implementation of the immunological platelet count on a hematology analyzer—the Abbott Cell-Dyn 4000®. Lab Hematol 1997; 3:125–128.

Bessman JD, Gilmer PR, Gardner FH. Improved classification of anemias MCV and RDW. Am J Clin Pathol 1983;80:322–326.

Bowen K, Procopio N, Wystepek E, et al. A preliminary evaluation of the Abbott Cell-Dyn 4000® automated flow cytometric flagging for platelet clumps by comparison to the Coulter STKS and manual blood smear on selected patient samples (abstr). Lab Hematol 1997;3:180.

Cell-Dyn 4000® System Operations Manual. PN 9140275-01 Abbott Diagnostics, Santa Clara, CA.

Centers for Disease Control and Prevention. 1997 revised guidelines for performing CD4+ T-cell determinations in persons infected with human immunodeficiency virus (HIV). MMWR 1997;46(No. RR-2):8–9.

Cornbleet J, Kessinger S. Evaluation of coulter S-Plus three-part differential in population with a high prevalence of abnormalities. Am J Clin Pathol 1985;84:620–626.

Coulter WH. High speed automatic blood cell counter and cell size analyzer. Proc Natl Electronics Conf 1956;12:1034.

Crossland-Taylor PJ. A device for counting small particles suspended in fluid through a tube. Nature 1953;171:37–38.

Dacie JV, Lewis SM. Appendix. In: Practical hematology. 7th ed. Edinburgh: Churchill Livingstone, 1991:543.

Davis BH, Bigelow NC, Curnette JT, et al. Neutrophil CD64 expression: potential diagnostic indicator of acute inflammation and therapeutic monitor of interferon-gamma therapy. Lab Hematol 1995;1:3–12.

d'Onofrio G, Zini G, Tommasi M, et al. Quantitative bone marrow analysis using the Abbott Cell-Dyn 4000® hematology analyzer. Lab Hematol 1997;3:146–153.

Dorner K, Schulze S, Reinhardt M, et al. Improved automated leukocyte counting and differential in newborns achieved by the haematology analyser Cell-Dyn 3500. Clin Lab Haematol 1995; 17:23–30.

England JM, Bashford CC, Hewer MG, et al. Simple method for automating the differential leukocyte count. Lancet 1975;i:492–493.

Givan AL. Flow cytometry first principles. New York: Wiley-Liss, 1992.

Glazier JR, Mazzella F, Roberts L, et al. Recovery of cultured leukemic blast cells by the Abbott Cell-Dyn 4000® automated hematology analyzer. Lab Hematol 1997; 3:138–145.

Groner W, Simson E. Integrating the analyzer into the hematology laboratory. In: Practical guide to modern hematology analyzers. Chichester, UK: Wiley & Sons, 1995: 188–197.

Groner W, Simson E. Practical guide to modern hematology analyzers. Chichester, UK: Wiley and Sons, 1995.

Hansen-Prus OC. The circulating blood cells as seen by dark-ground illumination. Am J Clin Pathol 1936;6:423–431.

Hubl W, Hauptlorenz S, Tlustos L, et al. Precision and accuracy of monocyte counting. Comparison of two hematology analyzers, the manual differential and flow cytometry. Am J Clin Pathol 1995;103:167–170.

Jones RG, Faust AM, Matthews RA, et al. Performance characteristics of the Cell-Dyn 3500 hematology analyzer on leukopenic whole blood samples. Lab Hematol 1996; 2:26–34.

Joyner RE, Brooks MJ. Evaluation of the automated leukocyte count and differential from the Cell-Dyn 3500 in sickle cell disease. Clin Lab Haematol 1995;17:329–333.

Kim YR, Yee M, Mehta S, et al. Simultaneous analysis of erythroblasts and white blood cell differential on a high throughput clinical instrument (abstr). Lab Hematol 1997; 3:181.

Mansberg HP, Saunders AM, Groner W. The Hemalog D white cell differential system. J Histochem Cytochem 1974;22:711–724.

Mullaney PF, Van Dilla MA, Coulter JR, et al. Cell sizing: a light scattering photometer for rapid volume determination. Rev Sci Instrum 1969;40:1029–1032.

National Committee for Clinical Laboratory Standards. Reference leukocyte differential count (proportional) and evaluation of instrumental methods; approved standard. NCCLS Document H20-A. Villanova, PA: NCCLS, 1992.

Rowan RM. Blood cell volume analysis—a new screening technology for the haematologist. London: Albert Clark and Company Limited, 1983.

Salzman GC, Crowell JM, Martin JC, et al. Cell classification by laser light scattering: identification and separation of unstained leukocytes. Acta Cytol 1975;19:374–377.

Sasche C, Henkel E. An evaluation of the Cell-Dyn 1700 haematology analyser: automated cell counting and three-part leucocyte differentiation. Clin Lab Haematol 1996;18:171–180.

Shapiro HM. Afterword. In: Practical flow cytometry. 2nd ed. New York: Wiley-Liss, 1988:307.

Shapiro HM. Practical flow cytometry. 2nd ed. New York: Wiley-Liss, 1988.

Sysmex SE-9000 Operator's Manual. No. 461-2455-9 Toa Medical Electronics Co Ltd, Kobe, 1994.

Terstappen LWMM, de Grooth BG, Visscher K, et al. Four parameter white blood cell differential counting based on light scattering measurements. Cytometry 1988; 9:39–43.

Van Dilla MA, Fulwyler MJ, Boone IU. Volume distribution and separation of normal human leukocytes. Proc Soc Exp Biol Med 1967;125:367.

Van Dilla MA, Trujillo TT, Mullaney PF, et al. Cell microfluorimetry; a method for rapid fluorescence measurement. Science 1969;163:1213.

von Behrens W. Particulate matter analyzing apparatus and method. U.S. Patent 4,710,021, 1987.

Wycherly PA, O'Shea MJ. Abridged differential leukocyte counts provided by a Coulter Channelyser in a routine haematology laboratory. J Clin Pathol 1987;31:271–274.

CHAPTER 8

Case Studies—Peripheral Blood

GENERAL COMMENTS

The following cases present examples of how information from the Cell-Dyn 3500 and 4000 systems can be utilized to detect the presence of abnormal cells within the scattergrams. It becomes increasingly clear that the instrument is able to detect different types of leukemic blasts. The blasts are characterized by size, lobularity, nuclear/cytoplasmic ratio, and ability to scatter polarized light. A normal peripheral blood is shown in Figure 8.0A and scatterplots in Figure 8.0B. In normal peripheral blood (Fig. 8.0B) the lymphocytes are blue, monocytes purple, neutrophils orange, eosinophils green, and basophils black.

The scattergrams that are advantageous for evaluation of blast cells includes the size (0°), fluorescent DNA (FL3); lobularity (90°), size (0°); and the size (0°), complexity (7°). The first scatterplot was used from the Cell-Dyn 4000® system; the last from the Cell-Dyn 3500 system. The lobularity (90°), size (0°) was used in both instruments. The blasts have a tendency to expand into and beyond the normal lymphocyte and monocyte populations. Since the diagnosis of acute leukemia is dependent on a unified multifaceted approach, automated instrumentation, as demonstrated here, should encompass a new facet that will be helpful in diagnosis.

NORMAL CONTROL: 43-year-old white male.

MEDICAL HISTORY: Good health without any acute or chronic illnesses.

PHYSICAL EXAMINATION: Within normal limits.

CELL-DYN 4000®

WBC (viability)	5.06×10^9/L (99.9%)
Hemoglobin	14.9 g/dL
Platelets	299×10^9/L
Neutrophils	2.59×10^9/L(51.2%)
Lymphocytes	1.95×10^9/L(38.5%)
Monocytes	0.363×10^9/L(7.18%)
Eosinophils	0.133×10^9/L(2.63%)
Basophils	0.025×10^9/L(0.489%)

The important scattergrams for detection of blasts include the size (0° light scatter) and fluorescent DNA (left) and the lobularity (90° light scatter) and size (0° right) (Fig. 8.0B). The analyzer indicated that 99.9% of the leukocytes were viable. Measurement of viability (permeability) is dependent on

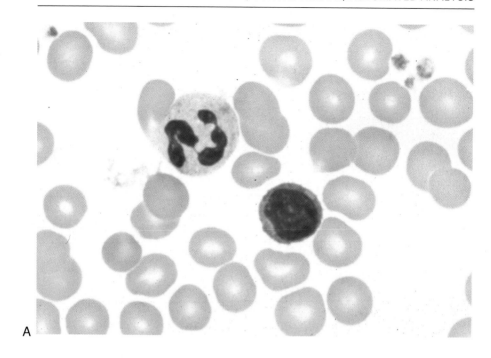

A

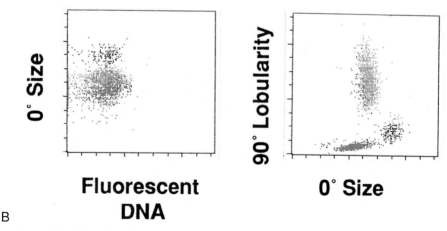

B

Figure 8.0. A. Peripheral blood showing normal cellular elements (× 1000). B. Showing scatterplots of normal peripheral blood. Size (0°), fluorescent DNA (FL3) scatterplot (left). Lobularity (90°), size (0°), scatterplot (right). Granulocytes (orange), lymphocytes (blue), monocytes (purple), eosinophils (green), basophils (black).

exclusion of propidium iodide, a fluorescent DNA stain, from a cell's nucleus by its intact cytoplasmic membrane. The left scattergram shows the monocytes (purple), granulocytes (orange), lymphocytes (blue), eosinophils (green), and basophils (black). Note that the right side of the scattergram is clear, indicating absence of nonviable cells. The right scattergram separates the cells by lobularity (90° light scatter) and size (0° light scatter). Note the location of the various cell types on these scattergrams. Blasts on the size (0° light scatter) and fluorescent DNA scattergram should appear in the monocytic (purple) region; however, if small (acute lymphoblastic leukemia [ALL] L1), they would be found in the lymphocyte (blue) region. Blasts on the lobularity (90° light scatter) and size (0° light scatter) are usually located below and to the right of the monocytes; however, monoblasts and notched or lobulated blasts may extend upward into the monocyte region.

CASE 1—ACUTE MYELOID LEUKEMIA

FAB M5A—ACUTE MONOBLASTIC LEUKEMIA, UNDIFFERENTIATED, THERAPY RELATED

PATIENT: 57-year-old white male.

CHIEF COMPLAINT: Cough, fever, night sweats, and blood-tinged sputum.

MEDICAL HISTORY: Patient diagnosed as poorly differentiated stage IV non-Hodgkin lymphoma in January 1986. Received multiple cycles of chemotherapy that included alkylating agents and topoisomerase inhibitors. Also received radiation therapy to the spine. Bone marrow 4 months previously was normal.

PHYSICAL EXAMINATION: Elevated temperature, rales right posterior lower thorax.

CELL-DYN 3500

WBC	3.01×10^9/L
Hemoglobin	9.76 g/dL
Platelets	18.7×10^9/L
Neutrophils	0.385×10^9/L (12.8%)
Lymphocytes	0.303×10^9/L (10.1%)
Monocytes	1.73×10^9/L (57.4%)
Eosinophils	0.021×10^9/L (0.71%)
Basophils	0.576×10^9/L (19.1%)
Suspect Flags	Immature grans/blasts

The analyzer results correlated reasonably well with those from the manual blood film examination. The analyzer classified the monocytic precursors as monocytes (57.4%), and flagged the presence of blasts. The manual differential count indicated 60% monoblasts and promonocytes (Fig. 8.1).

ADDITIONAL DATA: The marrow was hypercellular with 98% infiltra-

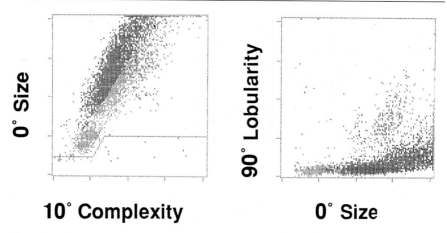

0° Size

10° Complexity

90° Lobularity

0° Size

Figure 8.1. Scattergram shows large population of blasts and promonocytes (purple); extending upward and to the right (left). Right scattergram demonstrates large blasts with slight upward extension indicating some clefting.

tion with large vacuolated blasts that were A-EST+, sensitive to fluoride; myeloperoxidase negative (MPEX−), and Sudan black B positive (SBB+) (Fig. 8.2).

Immunohistochemical stains revealed CD68+, antilysozyme strongly+, MPEX−. Immunostain to detect residual lymphoma CD20, CD3 were negative. Flow cytometric analysis: the cells were CD34+, CD13+, CD14−, CD33−, HLA-DR−, and CD3− indicating a population of immature progenitor cells. Interestingly, cytogenetics demonstrated changes compatible with the previous lymphoma in addition to therapy-induced abnormalities; 11q23, a topoisomerase inhibitor defect.

COMMENT: Therapy-related leukemic syndromes occur most frequently in long-term survivors of non-Hodgkin lymphoma, Hodgkin disease, ovarian cancer, multiple myeloma, small cell carcinoma of the lung, and gastrointestinal cancer who have been exposed to alkylating agents and radiation. The majority of these patients present with myelodysplastic features before developing frank acute leukemia. In 25% of all cases, there is an abrupt appearance of acute myeloid leukemia (AML) without the preleukemic phase. The FAB classification is difficult to define in most of these incidences because of multilineage involvement. Since monoblasts in the bone marrow accounted for more than 80% of the monocytic series, the

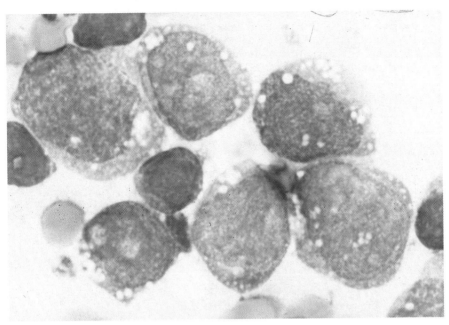

Figure 8.2. Bone marrow showing large, round and oval blasts with irregular nuclear membranes, nucleoli, scanty basophilic cytoplasm and vacuolated nuclei and cytoplasm (× 1000).

patient was classified as FAB M5a, which is seen in topoisomerase inhibitor treated patients.

The scattergram (Fig. 8.1) is dominated by a large population of cells (purple) occupying both the normal monocyte area and a greater area above, indicating the presence of very large blasts (size 0°, complexity 10° left). Note the expansion of blasts in lobularity 90°, size 0° with extension upward probably relating to clefted nuclei in some blasts. Bone marrow showed large oval blasts with sparse vacuolated basophilic cytoplasm. Occasionally, the blasts were indented and demonstrated vacuoles in the nucleus.

BIBLIOGRAPHY

Articles

Bredeson CN, Barnett MJ, Horsman DE, et al. Therapy-related acute myelogenous leukemia associated with 11q23 chromosomal abnormalities and topoisomerase II inhibitors: report of four additional cases and brief commentary. Leuk Lymphoma 1993;11:141–145.

Dorner K, Schulze S, Reinhardt M, et al. Improved automated leucocyte counting and differential in newborns achieved by the haematology analyser Cell Dyn 3500. Clin Lab Haematol 1995;17:23–30.

Fournier M, Gireau A, Chretien MC, et al. Laboratory evaluation of the Abbott Cell–Dyn 3500 5-part differential. Am J Clin Pathol 1996;105:286–292.

Hoffmann L, Moller P, Pedersen-Bjergaard J, et al. Therapy-related acute promyelocytic leukemia with t(15;17) (q22;q12) following chemotherapy with drugs targeting DNA topoisomerase II. Ann Oncol 1995;6:781–788.

Stark B, Jeison M, Shohat M, et al. Involvement of 11p15 and 3q21q26 in therapy-related myeloid leukemia (t-ML) in children. Cancer Genet Cytogenet 1994;75:11–22.

Vives-Corrons JL, Besson I, Jou JM, et al. Evaluation of the Abbott Cell-Dyn 3500 hematology analyzer in university hospital. Am J Clin Pathol 1996;105:553–559.

CASE 2—ACUTE EOSINOPHILIC LEUKEMIA

PATIENT: 21-year-old black female.

CHIEF COMPLAINT: Abdominal pain, rectal bleeding, myalgias, and fatigue.

MEDICAL HISTORY: Approximately 1 month prior to admission to the university hospital, the patient developed a fever and pruritic rash. Treated with steroids, but developed abdominal pain and rectal bleeding. Complete blood count revealed an eosinophilia of 59% (Fig. 8.3).

PHYSICAL EXAMINATION: Elevated temperature and pruritic rash.

HOSPITAL COURSE: Extensive connective tissue disease work up was instituted and found to be entirely negative. On the fourth hospital day the patient was found obtunded and incontinent. She was transferred to a medical intensive care unit for acute respiratory distress syndrome, but failed to respond and died. Postmortem examination revealed the immediate cause of death was disseminated intravascular coagulation (DIC) and diffuse alveolar damage with underlying cause of death being eosinophilic leukemia.

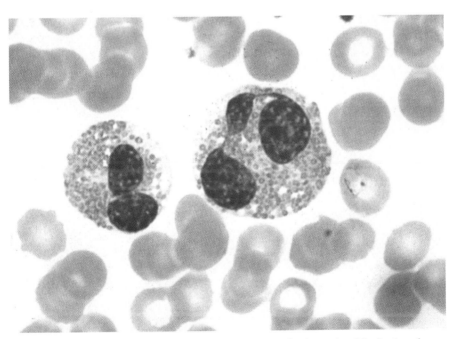

Figure 8.3. Peripheral blood showing eosinophils with vacuolization and maldistribution of granules. Note large eosinophil has three lobes (✕ 1000).

CELL-DYN 3500

WBC	19×10^9/L
Hemoglobin	11.7 g/dL
Platelets	264×10^9/L
Neutrophils	5.19×10^9/L (27%)
Lymphocytes	1.78×10^9/L (9.4%)
Monocytes	0.56×10^9/L (3%)
Eosinophils	11.3×10^9/L (59%)
Basophils	0.125×10^9/L (0.7%)

The analyzer results correlated with those from the manual blood film (Fig. 8.4).

ADDITIONAL DATA: The bone marrow at postmortem was hypercellular with 90% infiltration by eosinophils, immature eosinophilic precursors, and blasts. The M:E ratio was greater than 10:1.

Immunohistochemical stains revealed the following: MPEX strongly +, lysozyme strongly +, hemoglobin A+ on rare scattered clusters of nucleated red blood cells, factor VIII+ in megakaryocytes. Luna stain for eosinophils was positive. Electron microscopy revealed immature precursors and blasts

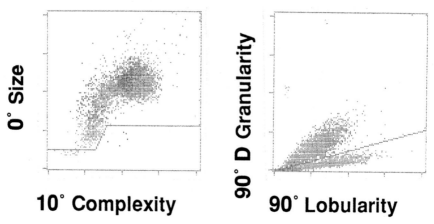

Figure 8.4. Left scattergram showing large population of eosinophils (green) extending to right of neutrophils (orange). Right scattergram demonstrates eosinophils' ability to depolarize light. Note extension of eosinophils extending toward origin, supporting the presence of some mononuclear eosinophils with both crystalline and non-crystalline granules.

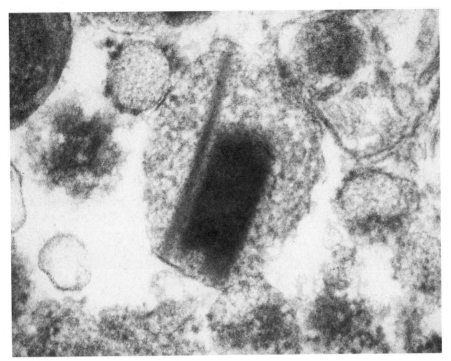

Figure 8.5. Electron micrograph shows crystalline structure within the granule, which acts as a tiny mirror depolarizing the light and separating eosinophils from the other granulocytes. The elongated extension on the side of the granule is considered abnormal. (× 100,000).

with eosinophilic granular crystalline structure (Fig. 8.5). Reverse transcripterase polymerase chain reaction (RT-PCR) on paraffin blocks for bcr rearrangement was negative. Autopsy revealed eosinophilic involvement of the heart, lungs, liver, spleen, thymus, and lymph nodes.

COMMENT: Eosinophilic leukemia is difficult to almost impossible to distinguish from the hypereosinophilic syndrome; however, the presence of immature forms invading tissue and infiltrating the bone marrow with associated involvement of hematologic parameters is strong evidence for a diagnosis of leukemia. The tissue damage occurs secondary to the release of major basic protein from the eosinophilic secondary granules. Confirmatory evidence requires demonstration of a clonal cytogenetic abnormality. Unfortunately, karyotypic analysis was not performed in this case.

The analyzer identifies eosinophils by the high 90° depolarized light scatter (granularity) signal produced by the granules of this cell type. The electron micrograph clearly shows the crystalline core within the granule that acts as a tiny mirror causing unique scatter of the laserlight and separation of eosinophils from other granulocytic cells. Since these eosinophils and eosinophilic precursors were more bizarre than normal eosinophils, an unusual pattern extending to the origin of the 90° D/90° scatterplot was observed. This was related to the fact that some of the eosinophilic precursors lacked lobularity and some contained mixtures of crystalline and noncrystalline granules.

BIBLIOGRAPHY

Articles

Schumacher HR, Cotelingam JD. Case 6—hypereosinophilic syndrome terminating in monocytic leukemia (AML 5a). In: Chronic leukemia: approach to diagnosis. New York: Igaku-Shoin, 1993:245–259.

Terstappen LWMM, de Grooth BG, Visscher K, et al. Four-parameter white blood cell differential counting based on light scattering measurements. Cytometry 1988;9:39–43.

Vives-Corrons JL, Besson I, Jou JM, et al. Evaluation of the Abbott Cell-Dyn 3500 hematology analyzer in university hospital. Am J Clin Pathol 1996;105:553–559.

Review Articles

Fauci AS, Harley JB, Roberts WC, et al. The idiopathic hypereosinophilic syndrome. Ann Intern Med 1982;97:78–92.

Keene P, Mendelow B, Pinto MR, et al. Abnormalities of chromosome 12p13 and malignant proliferation of eosinophils: a nonrandom association. Br J Haematol 1987;67:25–31.

Presentey B, Jerushalmy Z, Mintz U. Eosinophilic leukemia. Morphological, cytochemical and electron microscopic studies. J Clin Pathol 1979;32:261–271.

CASE 3—ACUTE MYELOID LEUKEMIA

FAB M0—ACUTE MYELOBLASTIC LEUKEMIA, MINIMALLY DIFFERENTIATED

PATIENT: 34-year-old white male.

CHIEF COMPLAINT: Fever, cough, sinus disease, and weight loss.

MEDICAL HISTORY: Several weeks prior to admission, the patient complained of malaise, fatigue, intermittent fever with night sweats, and lower back pain that did not respond to nonsteroidal antiinflammatory agents. Three weeks before admission, he developed an episode of acute sinusitis and acute bronchitis, which was treated with Unasyn with little improvement.

PHYSICAL EXAMINATION: Fever, no organomegaly.

CELL-DYN 3500

WBC	4.13×10^9/L
Hemoglobin	7.86 g/dL
Platelets	55.4×10^9/L
Neutrophils	0.473×10^9/L (11.5%)
Lymphocytes	2.19×10^9/L (53.1%)
Monocytes	1.04×10^9/L (25.3%)
Eosinophils	0.024×10^9/L (0.6%)
Basophils	0.40×10^9/L (9.6%)
Suspect Flags	DLTA
	IG/Bands
	Blast
	NRBC

This peripheral blood specimen in EDTA was referred to our laboratory over the weekend. The material was over 36 hours old when analyzed, but the analyzer still identified immature granulocytes/bands, blasts (Fig. 8.6), and nucleated red blood cells. The instrument showed a DELTA (DLTA) flag, which indicates a discrepancy between the white blood cell (WBC) impedance count (WIC), a total nucleated count, and WBC optical count (WOC), a gated optical count due to nucleated red blood cells (NRBC) being counted in the WIC, and NRBC being excluded from the WOC. In this case the instrument selected the correct count: the WOC.

ADDITIONAL DATA: The peripheral blood demonstrated occasional blast cells (Fig. 8.7). Less than 3% of the blasts reacted for MPEX, SBB, or NSE in the bone marrow.

Immunohistochemical stains on the bone marrow for CD68, antilysozyme, and MPEX were negative. Flow cytometric analysis on the bone marrow revealed that greater than 20% of the blasts were positive for CD13

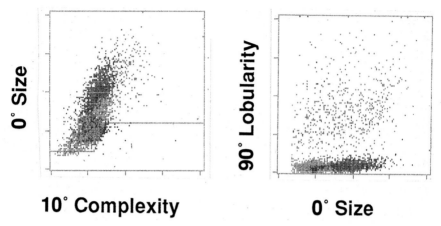

Figure 8.6. Scattergram shows cells extending upward (purple), scattered degenerating neutrophils (orange), incorrect basophil (blasts with low N/C ratio) analysis (black) and nucleated red blood cells (red) (left) (size 0°, complexity 10°). Right scattergram shows cells in blast region (purple) and large numbers of degenerating granulocytes (orange) (lobularity 90°, size 0°).

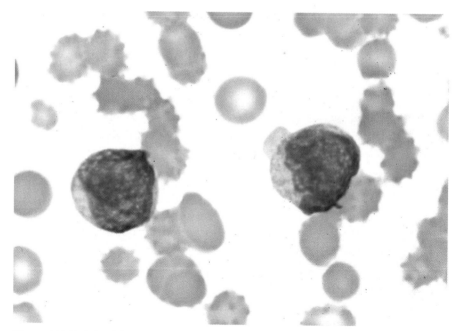

Figure 8.7. Peripheral blood showing blasts with oval, round, occasionally indented nuclei. Some of the blasts demonstrated nucleoli. The basophilic cytoplasm was scant to moderately abundant (× 1000).

and CD33. Interestingly, the CD7 and TdT were also positive; a finding present in some cases of FABM M0. The TdT is usually less positive than in ALL. Ultrastructural analysis of the MPEX-stained tissue may reveal reactivity present in the granules, the nuclear envelope, and the endoplasmic reticulum of these cells.

Cytogenetics revealed a normal male karyotype.

HOSPITAL COURSE: Bone marrow was performed and revealed a hypercellular marrow (F:C 5:95) that was replaced by blasts. The patient received high dose Ara-C with eventual complete remission.

COMMENT: The AML M0 is a relatively newly established FAB subtype whose diagnosis cannot be made on morphologic and cytochemical light-microscopy criteria alone. A case is defined as AML M0 when the MPEX/SBB is negative or less than 3%. Flow cytometric analysis reacts with at least one of the myeloid-specific antibodies (MPO, CD13, CD33), and lymphoid markers are negative (CD7 and TdT may be positive). Most cases express CD34, HLA-DR, and demonstrate a multidrug resistance phenotype. Ultrastructural MPEX may be used to establish the diagnosis. Differential diagnosis includes AUL, ALL, AML M5a, AML M7, and acute basophilic leukemia that can be clarified by flow cytometric analysis, cytochemical stains, and ultrastructural analysis. These patients have a very poor prognosis and many cases may relapse as monoblastic or megakaryocytic leukemia, suggesting orientation of M0 cells toward those lineages.

The scattergram (Fig. 8.6) (size 0°, complexity 10°, left) demonstrates an expansion of the monocyte area (purple) upward, representing the blast population. The black area represents the instrument's incorrect attempt to characterize the blasts with a low N/C ratio as basophils. The red area correctly identifies the presence of nucleated red blood cells. The (lobularity 90°, size 0°) scattergram (right) reveals the blasts (purple) extending along the X-axis. Note wide scatter of neutrophils (orange dots) due to break down over the delayed time period to analysis. Interestingly, the leukemic blasts seemed to retain fairly good morphology and probably viability.

BIBLIOGRAPHY

Articles

Cadwell FJ, Burns CP, Dick FR, et al. Minimally differentiated acute leukemia. Leuk Res 1993;17:199–208.

Cuneo A, Ferrant A, Michaux JL, et al. Cytogenetic profile of minimally differentiated (FAB M0) acute myeloid leukemia: correlation with clinicobiologic findings. Blood 1995;85:3688–3694.

Lee EJ, Pollak A, Leavitt RD, et al. Minimally differentiated acute nonlymphocytic leukemia: a distinct entity. Blood 1987;70:1400–1406.

Review Articles

Amadori S, Venditti A, Del Poeta G, et al. Minimally differentiated acute myeloid leukemia (AML M0): a distinct clinicobiologic entity with poor prognosis. Ann Hematol 1996;72:208–215.

Cheson BD, Cassileth PA, Head DR, et al. Report of the National Cancer Institute-sponsored workshop on definitions of diagnosis and response in acute myeloid leukemia. J Clin Oncol 1990;8:813–819.

Keung YK, Kaplan B, Douer D. Biphenotypic M0 acute myeloid leukemia with trisomy-4. Leuk Lymphoma 1994;14:181–184.

Taylor CG, Stasi R, Bastianelli C, et al. Diagnosis and classification of the acute leukemias: recent advances and controversial issues. Hematopathol Mol Hematol 1996;10:1–38.

CASE 4—ACUTE MYELOID LEUKEMIA

FAB M6B—ACUTE PURE RED CELL ERYTHROLEUKEMIA

PATIENT: 47-year-old black male.

CHIEF COMPLAINT: Fatigue, malaise, and weight loss.

MEDICAL HISTORY: Patient had a past medical history of renal transplant. He had been given continuous cyclosporine until 1 year ago, when he was diagnosed with refractory anemia with ringed sideroblasts (RARS).

PHYSICAL EXAMINATION: Splenomegaly.

HOSPITAL COURSE: A bone marrow (Fig. 8.8) was performed and revealed large numbers of erythroid precursors. Many of these were proerythroblasts. A diagnosis of acute erythroleukemia M6b was established. The patient received a 3-week course of arabinosylcytosine (Ara-C) and daunorubicin. Follow up bone marrow revealed a decrease in hematopoiesis, but the proerythroblasts remained. Analysis of the peripheral blood revealed circulating viable blasts (Fig. 8.9).

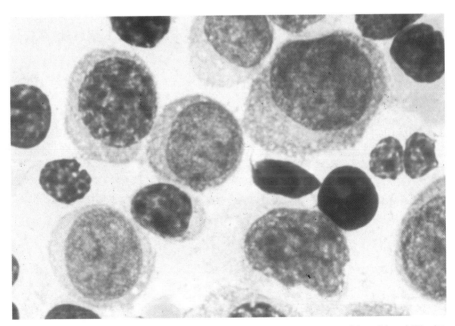

Figure 8.8. Bone marrow showing numerous proerythroblasts compatible with a M6b. (× 1000).

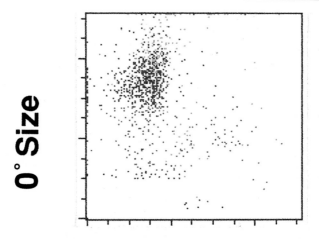

Fluorescent DNA

Figure 8.9. Scattergram of a buffy coat demonstrating blast cells (purple) by size and fluorescent DNA. The viability is determined by the cell's ability to exclude propidium iodide from staining the nucleus. The viability in this specimen was 92.0% indicating that the blast cells were unaffected by the chemotherapy.

CELL-DYN 4000® LABORATORY WORKSHEET*
(POST TREATMENT)

WBC (Viability)	0.781×10^9/L (92.0%)
Hemoglobin	9.5 g/dL
Platelets	9.37×10^9/L
Neutrophils	0.178×10^9/L (22.9%)
Bands	0.004×10^9/L (0.5%)
IG	0.02×10^9/L (2.6%)
Blasts	0.258×10^9/L (33.1%)
Monocytes	0.151×10^9/L (19.3%)
Eosinophils	0.024×10^9/L (3.1%)
Basophils	0.00×10^9/L (0.00%)
Lymphocytes	0.095×10^9/L (12.1%)
Variant Lymphs	0.050×10^9/L (6.43%)
Suspect Flags	Band
	IG
	Blast
	Varlym

*For laboratory use only.

The analyzer results correlated reasonably well with the manual differential that revealed 23% blasts, bands, immature granulocytes, and heavily vacuolated monocytes. The blasts and unusual monocytes were most likely responsible for the variant lymph flag.

ADDITIONAL DATA: The bone marrow at diagnosis revealed a F:C ratio of 10:90. The erythroid elements predominated with many proerythroblasts (Fig. 8.8) compatible with a M6b. Cytochemical stains revealed PAS positivity: blush (mature erythroid elements), block (proerythroblasts).
Flow cytometric analysis was not helpful. This has been our experience with other erythroleukemias. Glycophorin does not effectively label proerythroblasts.
Immunohistochemical stain for hemoglobin A revealed that many of the proerythroblasts and erythroid elements were positive.

COMMENT: The American Society of Hematopathology and World Health Organization has recently adopted our criteria for erythroleukemia. FAB M6 (Di Guglielmo's syndrome) has been designated FAB M6a, and pure erythroleukemia (Di Guglielmo's disease) has been designated M6b. FAB M6a is characterized by myeloblastic predominance, less toxic exposure, minor karyotypic abnormalities, better response to therapy, and longer survival. FAB M6b is characterized by proerythroblastic predominance, more toxic exposure, major karyotypic abnormalities, poor response to therapy and short survival. Proliferation markers Ki-67 and proliferating cell nuclear antigen (PCNA) are significantly higher in FAB M6b that correlates with their poor survival. An additional group M6c also exists, which represents a combination of M6a and M6b.

As in patients receiving other immunosuppressants, those patients treated with cyclosporine are at increased risk for development of lymphomas and other malignancies, particularly those of the skin. Such patients should also be monitored for development of acute leukemia.

The scattergram demonstrated viability after intensive therapy (size 0°, fluorescent DNA, left). Note the blasts (purple) are quite large. This viability plot scattergram with the indicated percentage of viable cells has obvious potential for monitoring the effectiveness of chemotherapy on the leukemic population.

BIBLIOGRAPHY

Articles

Cuneo A, Van Orshoven A, Michaux JL, et al. Morphologic, immunologic, and cytogenetic studies in erythroleukemia: evidence for multilineage involvement and identification of two distinct cytogenetic-clinicopathological types. Br J Haematol 1990;75:346–354.
Davey FR, Abraham N Jr, Brunetto VL, et al. Morphologic characteristics of erythro-

leukemia (acute myeloid leukemia; FAB M6): a CALGB study. Am J Hematol 1995;49:29–38.

Garand R, Duchayne E, Blanchard D, et al. Minimally differentiated erythroleukaemia (AML M6 "variant"): a rare subset of AML distinct from AML M6. Groupe Francais d'Hematologie Cellulaire. Br J Haematol 1995;90:868–875.

Kowal-Vern A, Cotelingam JD, Schumacher HR. The prognostic significance of proerythroblasts in acute erythroleukemia. Am J Clin Pathol 1992;98(1):34–40.

Laskin WB, Cotelingam JD, Duval-Arnould B, et al. Erythroleukemia in a child: value of immunocytochemistry and transmission electron microscopy in its diagnosis. Am J Pediatr Hematol Oncol 1985;7:99–103.

Olopade OI, Thangavelu M, Larson RA, et al. Clinical, morphologic, and cytogenetic characteristics of 26 patients with acute erythroblastic leukemia. Blood 1992;80:2873–2882.

Siebert R, Jhanwar S, Brown K, et al. Familial acute myeloid leukemia and Di Guglielmo syndrome. Leukemia 1995;9:1091–1094.

Review Article

Grignani F, Testa U, Fagioli M, et al. Oncogenes and erythroid differentiation. Semin Can Biol 1994;5:125–135.

CASE 5—ACUTE MYELOID LEUKEMIA

FAB M1—ACUTE MYELOBLASTIC LEUKEMIA WITHOUT MATURATION

PATIENT: 76-year-old white female.

CHIEF COMPLAINT: Fever associated with dry cough.

MEDICAL HISTORY: Patient's health had been relatively good up until present episode.

PHYSICAL EXAMINATION: Elevated temperature, rales in left posterior lower thorax.

HOSPITAL COURSE: Peripheral blood evaluation revealed a large number of blast cells (Fig. 8.10). Bone marrow examination including cytochemistries, immunohistochemistries, and flow cytometric analysis established a diagnosis of FAB M1. The patient was treated with Ara-C and daunorubicin that produced a severe pancytopenia. She was supported with blood transfusions and GM-CSF.

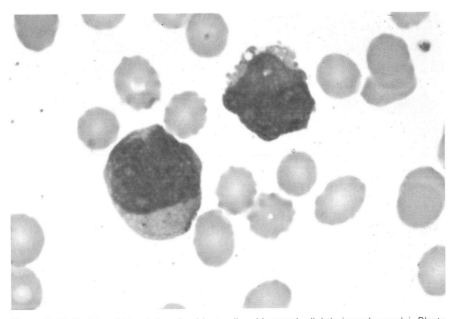

Figure 8.10. Peripheral blood showing blast cells with round, slightly irregular nuclei. Blasts have scanty, bubbly to moderate basophilic cytoplasm. Note prominent, multiple nucleoli (× 1000).

CELL-DYN 3500

WBC	$31.8 \times 10^9/L$
Hemoglobin	$6.8 \times g/dL$
Platelets	$46.8 \times 10^9/L$
Neutrophils	$0.113 \times 10^9/L$ (0.36%)
Lymphocytes	$3.46 \times 10^9/L$ (10.9%)
Monocytes	$26.4 \times 10^9/L$ (83.1%)
Eosinophils	$0.01 \times 10^9/L$ (0.03%)
Basophils	$1.81 \times 10^9/L$ (5.68%)
Suspect Flags	Variant lymphs/Blast Diff (NLMEB)

The analyzer results correlated with the manual blood film examination. The manual differential revealed 91% blasts, 8% lymphocytes, 1% monocytes, and 1% nucleated red blood cells. The analyzer flagged the blasts as variant lymphs/blasts and placed them into the monocyte channel (83.1%) and basophil channel (5.68%)—the sum of which equals 88.78%; very close to the manual blast differential! The analyzer revealed an expansion in the monocytic area (purple) in both the depicted scattergrams (Fig. 8.11). Note the red dotted areas that represent nucleated red blood cells noted on the manual differential.

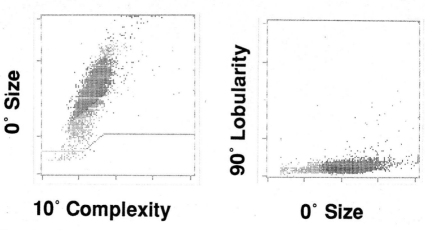

Figure 8.11. Scattergram of peripheral blood containing large numbers of blasts. Note the expansion of cells within the monocyte area (purple). Also, observe the events in the nucleated red blood cells region (red).

ADDITIONAL DATA: The marrow demonstrated 100% cellularity. It was composed of predominantly myeloid appearing blasts without differentiation similar to those in the peripheral blood.

Cytochemical analysis revealed MPEX+, SBB+, B-EST−, C-EST (CAE+, A-EST−).

Flow cytometric analysis performed on the peripheral blood demonstrated an acute myeloid leukemia pattern with CD13+, CD33+, HLA-DR+, and CD34−.

COMMENT: Acute myeloblastic leukemia without maturation, FAB AML M1 is characterized by a predominance of myeloblasts in the bone marrow that exceed 90%. Less than 10% of the marrow granulocytic cells show evidence of maturation to promyelocytes or beyond. FAB AML M1 must be distinguished from ALL L2, acute monoblastic leukemia FAB AML M5a, acute megakaryocytic leukemia FAB AML M7, and acute basophilic leukemia. These leukemias can be separated by cytochemical, immunohistochemical stains, and ultrastructural studies.

The scattergrams generated by the Cell-Dyn 3500 show expansion of the monocytic population (purple), which represents the large blast population. The large size of the blasts (purple) are represented by the left scatterplot (size 0°, and complexity 10°). The increased size of the blasts is also noted on the lobularity 90° and size 0° scattergram, right. Note that the blasts (purple) extend far to the right and do not extend upward, which would indicate cleaving or lobularity. The diff (NLMEB) flag appears because default thresholds were used to separate these cell types.

BIBLIOGRAPHY

Articles

Barnard DR, Kalousek DK, Wiersma SR, et al. Morphologic, immunologic, and cytogenetic classification of acute myeloid leukemia and myelodysplastic syndrome in childhood: a report from the Children's Cancer Group. Leukemia 1996;10:5–12.

Boban D, Sucic M, Markovic-Glamocak M, et al. Correlation of morphological FAB classification and immunophenotyping: value in recognition of morphological, cytochemical and immunological characteristics of mixed leukaemias. Eur J Cancer 1993;29A:1167–1172.

Bruno A, Del Poeta G, Venditti A, et al. Diagnosis of acute myeloid leukemia and system Coulter VCS. Haematologica 1994;79:420–428.

Del Poeta G, Stasi R, Venditti A, et al. Prognostic value of cell marker analysis in de novo acute myeloid leukemia. Leukemia 1994;8:388–394.

Kurec AS, Cruz VE, Barrett D, et al. Immunophenotyping of acute leukemias using paraffin-embedded tissue sections. Am J Clin Pathol 1990;93:502–509.

Lauria F, Raspadori D, Ventura MA, et al. The presence of lymphoid-associated antigens in adult acute myeloid leukemia is devoid of prognostic relevance. Stem Cells 1995;13:428–434.

Poirel H, Rack K, Delabesse E, et al. Incidence and characterization of MLL gene (11q23) rearrangements in acute myeloid leukemia M1 and M5. Blood 1996;

87:2496–2505.

Terstappen LW, Konemann S, Safford M, et al. Flow cytometric characterization of acute myeloid leukemia. Part 1. Significance of light scattering properties. Leukemia 1991;5:315–321.

Trecca D, Longo L, Biondi A, et al. Analysis of p53 gene mutations in acute myeloid leukemia. Am J Hematol 1994;46:304–309.

Wells SJ, Bray RA, Stempora LL, et al. CD117/CD34 expression in leukemic blasts. Am J Clin Pathol 1996;106:192–195.

Review Articles

Brunning RD, McKenna RW. Acute leukemias. In: Atlas of tumor pathology: tumors of the bone marrow. Fascicle 9. Washington, DC: AFIP, 1994:19–142.

Rohatiner A, Lister TA. Acute myelogenous leukemia in adults. In: Henderson ES, Lister TA, Greaves MF. Leukemia. 6th ed. Philadelphia: WB Saunders, 1996:479–512.

CASE 6—ACUTE MYELOID LEUKEMIA

FAB M4Eo—ACUTE MYELOMONOCYTIC LEUKEMIA WITH IN-CREASED MARROW EOSINOPHILS

PATIENT: 35-year-old white male.

CHIEF COMPLAINT: Fatigue, fever, and swollen gums.

MEDICAL HISTORY: Patient was in excellent health until his present illness.

PHYSICAL EXAMINATION: Elevated temperature, gingival hyperplasia, slight hepatosplenomegaly.

CELL-DYN 3500

WBC	28.4×10^9/L
Hemoglobin	9.74 g/dL
Platelets	40.3×10^9/L
Neutrophils	1.53×10^9/L (5.38%)
Lymphocytes	3.21×10^9/L (11.3%)
Monocytes	17.2×10^9/L (60.5%)
Eosinophils	0.344×10^9/L (1.21%)
Basophils	6.13×10^9/L (21.6%)
Suspect Flags	Blast

The analyzer correctly identified the presence of blast cells. The blast cells were classified in the monocyte and basophil category which added to 82.1%. Interestingly, the manual differential revealed 56% blasts and 27% monocytes, which totaled to 83%. Also, 4% basophils were observed (Fig. 8.12).

ADDITIONAL DATA: The bone marrow was hypercellular with 90% infiltration with large numbers of blasts. The percentage of myeloblasts, promonocytes, and monoblasts exceeded 30%. Both immature granulocytic and monocytic lineages accounted for more than 20% of the nucleated marrow cells. Eosinophils with basophilic granules were observed.

Cytochemical studies on the marrow revealed MPEX+, SBB+, B-EST+, A-EST+, CAE+, C-EST (CAE+, A-EST+) with A-EST sensitive to Fl. Eosinophils CAE+ and PAS+. Flow cytometric analysis demonstrated HLA-DR+, CD13+, CD34+, CD33+, and CD71+. Cytogenetic analysis revealed inv (16) (p13q22).

COMMENT: FAB M4Eo accounts for approximately 15 to 30% of cases of FAB AML M4 with increased abnormal eosinophils in the bone marrow (greater than 3%). A variable number of eosinophils show large misshapen basophilic granules that lack the normal crystalline structure of eosinophilic

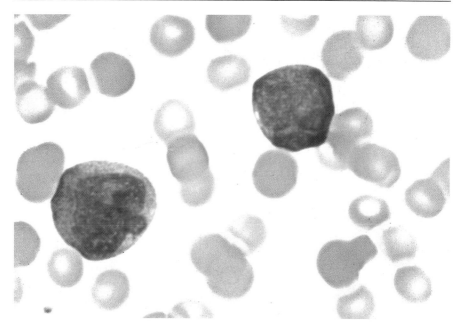

Figure 8.12. Peripheral blood exhibiting large numbers of blast cells. Blast in upper right shows high nuclear-cytoplasmic ratio with oval shaped nucleus (myeloblastic morphology). Blast, lower left reveals indented, clefted nucleus (monoblastic morphology) with moderate amounts of slightly basophilic cytoplasm (× 1000).

granules. Unlike normal eosinophils, the granules react with CAE and PAS. In most cases, as in this case, the increased eosinophil counts were not re-flected in the blood. Of interest in this case would be how such abnormal eosinophils would handle 90° depolarized light scatter (granularity). Since normal eosinophils contain crystalline structure within their granules that markedly depolarizes light more than granulocytes, such abnormal eosinophils lacking crystalline granular structure would be expected to be categorized in the granulocytic area (orange) on the granularity (90° depo-larized) versus lobularity (90°) analysis.

The scattergram is dominated by the presence of a large population of blasts (monoblasts, myeloblasts) that were placed in the monocytic category (purple) and flagged as blast (Fig. 8.13). The analyzer's attempt to classify some of the blasts resulted in these being categorized as basophils (black) (left scattergram). The scattergram on the right shows the separation of eosinophils and granulocytes by utilizing the granularity (90° depolarized) versus lobularity (90°) light scatter of the instrument. The abnormal eosinophils of M4Eo, without crystalline granular structure, would be ex-pected to fall below the line into the granulocytic (orange) area. The reader should also refer to Case 2—Acute Eosinophilic Leukemia (Chapter 9) for

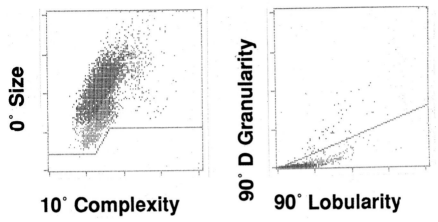

Figure 8.13. Scattergram shows large population of cells extending upward in the monocytic area (purple). Also, note some of the blasts with a lower N/C ratio were classified as basophils (black) (left). Normal eosinophils are demonstrated in green above the line (right). Abnormal eosinophils would be expected to extend toward and below the line in the granulocytic region (orange) due to lack of crystalline structure in their granules.

more information concerning the analyzer's attempt to classify abnormal eosinophils.

BIBLIOGRAPHY

Articles

Abruzzo LV, Jaffe ES, Cotelingam JD, et al. T-cell lymphoblastic lymphoma with eosinophilia associated with subsequent myeloid malignancy. Am J Surg Pathol 1992;16:236–245.

Creutzig U, Niederbiermann G, Ritter J, et al. Prognostic significance of eosinophilia in acute myelomonocytic leukemia in relation to induction treatment. Hamatologie und Bluttransfusion 1990;33:226–232.

Dengler R, Walther JU, Emmerich B. Trisomy 21 as the sole clonal aberration in a patient with acute myelomonocytic leukemia with abnormal bone marrow eosinophils and extramedullary involvement. Ann Hematol 1994;68:93–95.

Haferlach T, Gassmann W, Loffler H, et al. Clinical aspects of acute myeloid leukemias of the FAB types M3 and M4Eo. The AML Cooperative Group. Ann Hematol 1993;66:165–170.

Haferlach T, Winkemann M, Loffler H, et al. The abnormal eosinophils are part of the leukemic cell population in acute myelomonocytic leukemia with abnormal eosinophils (AML M4Eo) and carry the pericentric inversion 16: a combination of May-Grunwald-Giemsa staining and fluorescence in situ hybridization. Blood 1996;87:2459–2463.

Hebert J, Cayuela JM, Daniel MT, et al. Detection of minimal residual disease in acute myelomonocytic leukemia with abnormal marrow eosinophils by nested polymerase chain reaction with allele specific amplification. Blood 1994;84:2291–2296.

Monohan BP, Rector JT, Liu PP, et al. Clinical aspects of expression of inversion 16 chromosomal fusion transcript CBFB/MYH11 in acute myelogenous leukemia subtype M1 with abnormal bone marrow eosinophilia. Leukemia 1996;10:1653–1654.

Tasaka T, Nagai M, Bando S et al. Unbalanced translocation (1;7) and inversion 16 in a patient with acute myelocytic leukemia. Leuk Res 1993;17:699–701.

Review Articles

Brunning RD, McKenna RW. Acute leukemias. In: Brunning RD, McKenna RW. Atlas of tumor pathology: tumors of the bone marrow. Fascicle 9. Washington, DC: AFIP, 1994:53–56.

Drinkard LC, Waggoner S, Stein RN, et al. Acute myelomonocytic leukemia with abnormal eosinophils presenting as an ovarian mass: a report of two cases and a review of the literature. Gynecol Oncol 1995;56:307–311.

Liu PP, Hajra A, Wijmenga C, et al. Molecular pathogenesis of the chromosome 16 inversion in the M4Eo subtype of acute myeloid leukemia. Blood 1995;85:2289–2302.

CASE 7—ACUTE LYMPHOBLASTIC LEUKEMIA

T-CELL LYMPHOBLASTIC LEUKEMIA-LYMPHOMA

PATIENT: 52-year-old white male.

CHIEF COMPLAINT: Fever, night sweats, and large glands.

MEDICAL HISTORY: Prior to the present illness, the patient was in relatively good health.

PHYSICAL EXAMINATION: Elevated temperature, massive lymphadenopathy, and hepatosplenomegaly. No neurological abnormalities were detected.

CELL-DYN 4000®

WBC (Viability)	25.5×10^9/L (97.3%)
Hemoglobin	17.0 g/dL
Platelets	55.4×10^9/dL

The analyzer produced an invalid data flag, but correctly identified large numbers of variant lymphs (flagged) and blasts (flagged).

The manual differential revealed 64% lymphocytes, 6% blasts, 20% neutrophils, 3% bands, 2% eosinophils, and 5% monocytes (Fig. 8.14).

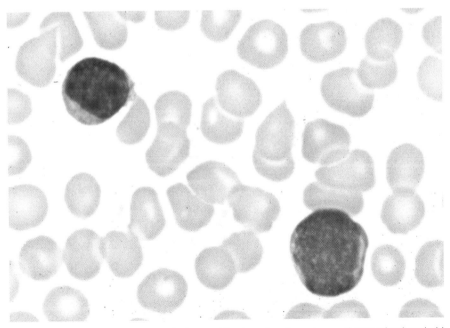

Figure 8.14. Peripheral blood revealed a combination of mature abnormal appearing lymphoid cells and lymphoblasts. Both showed slight convolutions in the nuclei. The nucleoli were inconspicuous in the blasts (× 1000).

The scattergram showed an expansion of the lymphoid (blue) population (Fig. 8.15).

ADDITIONAL DATA: Lymph node aspirate revealed numerous lymphoblastic cells that were consistent with a T-cell lymphoblastic leukemia-lymphoma. TdT was markedly positive. Immunohistochemistry revealed cytoplasmic CD3+ and CD43+. Flow cytometric analysis showed CD3+, CD5+, CD7+, and CD19+. The marrow demonstrated a F:C ratio of 2:98. Forty to 50% of the marrow was replaced by an interstitial lymphoid infiltrate consisting of immature cells with large convoluted nuclei, fine chromatin, and inconspicuous nucleoli, compatible with lymphoblasts. Cytochemical stains showed granular PAS+, AP focal unipolar positivity, and strong TdT positivity.

Immunohistochemical stains of the bone marrow revealed that most of the blasts were positive for CD3. Flow cytometric analysis on the bone marrow revealed the abnormal lymphoid cells to be CD2+, CD3+, CD5+, CD7+, and CD19+. The presence of the B-cell marker on a T cell lymphoblastic-leukemia/lymphoma is unusual. Nevertheless, Uckun et al. have shown that such patients treated with Children's Cancer Group protocols have good treatment outcomes.

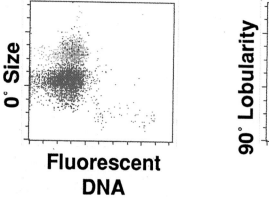

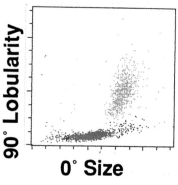

Figure 8.15. Scattergram shows expansion of abnormal lymphoid elements in all directions (blue) (left). This is also depicted in right scattergram. Note extension to right (purple) which represents blasts and variant lymphocytes.

HOSPITAL COURSE: The patient was treated with Ara-C, cytoxan, antibiotics, and supportive care. There was a dramatic decrease in the size of his massive lymphadenopathy. The WBC rose strikingly to 57×10^9/L with predominately convoluted lymphocytes.

CELL-DYN 4000® LABORATORY WORKSHEET

WBC (Viability)	68.7×10^9/L (98.3%)
Hemoglobin	$9.06 \times$ g/dL
Platelets	11×10^9/L
Neutrophils	12.1×10^9/L (17.6%)
Lymphocytes	53.7×10^9/L (78.2%)
Monocytes	0.05×10^9/L (0.07%)
Eosinophils	0.01×10^9/L (0.02%)
Variant Lymphs	1.07×10^9/L (1.56%)
Blasts	1.82×10^9/L (2.65%)
Suspect Flags	Blast
	Variant Lymphs

The patient developed respiratory disease, renal failure, disseminated intravascular, coagulation, and tumor lysis syndrome. He expired 14 days from the time of admission.

COMMENT: The incidence of bone marrow involvement by lymphoblastic lymphoma is 50 to 60%. The bone marrow may be the primary tissue available for examination in patients presenting with a mediastinal mass without peripheral lymphadenopathy. The histologic and cytologic features of lymphoblastic lymphoma are identical to those of acute lymphoblastic leukemia. The distinction is usually based on the percentage of lymphoblasts in the marrow at the time of diagnosis. If greater than 30% of the marrow cells are lymphoblasts, a designation of acute lymphoblastic leukemia is usually established. Since lymphoblastic lymphoma frequently involves marrow with leukemic-like cells, the term lymphoblastic leukemia-lymphoma has been used in cases of ALL with mass disease and T-cell immunophenotype. Seventy percent of cases of lymphoblastic lymphoma express T-cell immunophenotype, whereas, 30% exhibit a B-cell precursor immunophenotype.

The interesting finding in this patient was the dramatic rise in the malignant lymphocytes in the peripheral blood. These undoubtedly came from the shrinking lymph nodes. Also, of interest was the finding that these cells demonstrated 98.3% viability, indicating resistance to the chemotherapy!

The scattergram is dominated by a large expanded population of abnormal lymphocytes (blue) (left). This abnormal population is expanded in the right scattergram in both directions along the X-axis indicating small and large abnormal lymphoid elements.

BIBLIOGRAPHY

Articles

Abruzzo LV, Jaffe ES, Cotelingam JD, et al. T-cell lymphoblastic lymphoma with eosinophilia associated with subsequent myeloid malignancy. Am J Surg Pathol 1992;16:236–245.

Hasui K, Sato E, Sakae K, et al. Immunohistological quantitative analysis of S100 protein-positive cells in T-cell malignant lymphomas, especially in adult T-cell leukemia/lymphomas. Pathol Res Pract 1992;188:484–489.

Janssen JW, Ludwig WD, Sterry W, et al. SIL-TAL1 deletion in T-cell acute lymphoblastic leukemia. Leukemia 1993;7:1204–1210.

Kikuchi A, Hayashi Y, Kobayashi S, et al. Clinical significance of TAL1 gene alteration in childhood T-cell acute lymphoblastic leukemia and lymphoma. Leukemia 1993;7:933–938.

Osada H, Emi N, Ueda R, et al. Genuine CD7 expression in acute leukemia and lymphoblastic lymphoma. Leuk Res 1990;14:869–877.

Riopel M, Dickman PS, Link MP, et al. MIC2 analysis in pediatric lymphomas and leukemias. Hum Pathol 1994;25:396–399.

Shikano T, Arioka H, Kobayashi R, et al. Acute lymphoblastic leukemia and non-Hodgkin's lymphoma with mediastinal mass—a study of 23 children; different disorders or different stages? Leuk Lymphoma 1994;13:161–167.

Uckun FM, Gaynon P, Sather H, et al. Clinical features and treatment outcome of children with biphenotypic CD2+, CD19+ acute lymphoblastic leukemia: a Children's Cancer Group Study. Blood 1997;89:2488–2493.

Review Articles

Friedman HD, Inman DA, Hutchison RE, et al. Concurrent invasive thymoma and T-cell lymphoblastic leukemia and lymphoma. A case report with necropsy findings and literature review of thymoma and associated hematologic neoplasm. Am J Clin Pathol 1994;101:432–437.

Spigland N, Di Lorenzo M, Youssef S, et al. Malignant thymoma in children: a 20-year review. J Pediatr Surgery 1990;25:1143–1146.

CASE 8—ACUTE LYMPHOBLASTIC LEUKEMIA

FAB ALL L2—T-CELL ALL

PATIENT: 15-year-old white male.

CHIEF COMPLAINT: Tiredness, fatigue, lethargy.

MEDICAL HISTORY: In relatively good health up until present illness.

PHYSICAL EXAMINATION: Generalized lymphadenopathy, hepato-splenomegaly.

CELL-DYN 4000® LABORATORY WORKSHEET

WBC (Viability)	130×10^9/L (87.3%)
Hemoglobin	12.4 g/dL
Platelets	39.5×10^9/L
Neutrophils	3.96×10^9/L (3.06%)
IG	0.16×10^9/L (0.12%)
Lymphocytes	101×10^9/L (78.1%)
Monocytes	2.26×10^9/L (1.74%)
Eosinophils	1.14×10^9/L (0.87%)
Basophils	0.22×10^9/L (0.17%)
Variant Lymphs	15×10^9/L (11.6%)
Blasts	5.65×10^9/L (4.36%)
Suspect Flags	IG
	Blast
	Variant Lymphs

The differential was difficult in that many bizarre atypical lymphocytes and blast cells were present. The manual differential revealed 22% lymphocytes, 38% atypical lymphocytes, 33% blasts, 2% monocytes, 4% neutrophils and immature granulocytes, and 1% eosinophils (Fig. 8.16). The analyzer had difficulty correctly sorting out the spectrum of lymphoid cells, but correctly flagged blasts, variant lymphocytes, and immature granulocytes. A distinct population of small lymphoid cells with little or no cytoplasm and markedly hyperchromatic nuclei with frequent prominent nuclear convolutions were noted (Fig. 8.17).

ADDITIONAL DATA: The marrow was markedly cellular with numerous large lymphoblasts. Some of the blasts demonstrated folded, clefted, irregular nuclei. Nucleoli were prominent in some of the blast cells. The small lymphoid cells noted in the peripheral blood were also observed.

Cytochemistry on the bone marrow revealed PAS+ with large granules, MPEX−, SBB−, B-EST−, A-EST+, TdT+.

Flow cytometric analysis on the bone marrow revealed the abnormal lymphoid cells to be CD7+, CD2+, CD5+, CD3+, and CD13+ (Myeloid marker).

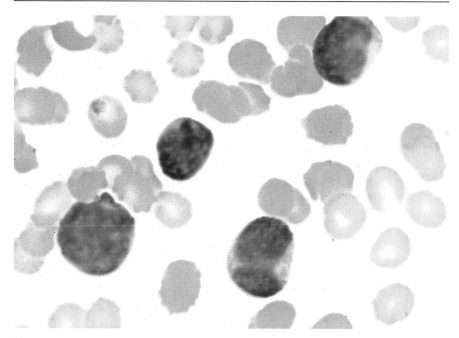

Figure 8.16. Peripheral blood showed large blasts with high nuclear/cytoplasmic ratio, and atypical bizarre lymphoid cells. Small hyperchromatic convoluted blasts were also noted. Some of the lymphoid cells revealed vacuolated basophilic cytoplasm (× 1000).

Cytogenetics revealed 46, XY, ins (10;11)(p12;q13q23)[16]46, XY[4]. FISH with an 11 paint probe confirmed ins (10;11).

MLL gene was discovered to be rearranged by Southern blot analysis.

HOSPITAL COURSE: The patient was treated with adriamycin, vincristine, asparaginase, and prednisone. At day 14, the marrow revealed large numbers of residual blast cells supporting a highly resistant leukemia.

COMMENT: Approximately 15% of patients with ALL are of the T-cell type. The lymphoblasts usually express one or more pan-T-cell monoclonal antibodies such as CD2, CD5, and CD7. Surface CD3 which was present on 93% of the lymphoid cells in this case is commonly lacking on the cell surface in T-cell ALL. T-cell ALLs are fairly uniformly distributed at early, intermediate, and mature thymocyte stages, but phenotypic aberrancy is fairly common. T-cell ALL may be either FAB L1 or L2, however, some studies have shown a predominance of L2. In the majority of cases a variable number of distinct small cells with little or no cytoplasm and markedly hyperchromatic nuclei, often with prominent nuclear convolutions are seen in the

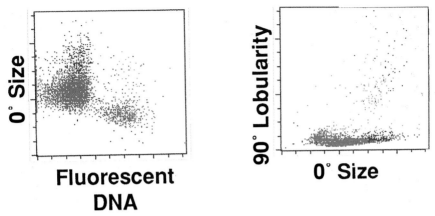

Figure 8.17. Scattergrams show an expansion of the lymphoid population (blue). The left scattergram depicts the non-viable lymphoid cells (blue) to lower right. The right scattergram shows purple dots to extreme right representing the blast population and left representing the small lymphoid cells with a high nuclear-cytoplasmic ratio and hypercrhomatic nuclei.

blood and bone marrow. These unique small cells always occur with a predominant population of larger leukemic blasts.

Studies have shown a fairly uniform distribution of T-cell ALL at early, intermediate, and mature thymocyte stages, with phenotypic aberrancy as observed in this case relatively common.

The important breakpoint in this patient's karyotype is the 11q23 since it was associated with disruption of the MLL gene. Such a disruption confers a poor prognosis, as observed in the treatment response noted in this case.

The scattergram is dominated by a large expanded population of abnormal lymphocytes (blue) that includes blasts, atypical, bizarre, and small hyperchromatic convoluted lymphocytes (left) (Fig. 8.17).

Note that in the right scattergram, the lymphoid population (blue) is greatly expanded in both directions along the X-axis indicating both the small and larger lymphoid cells. The extension upward is related to the lobularity of some of the lymphocytes. The purple areas to the extreme right represent blast cells, since it is not in the area for monocytes. This is the area where blast cells appear in the lobularity (90°)/size (0°) scattergram.

More on T-ALL can be found in Case 7 in this chapter.

BIBLIOGRAPHY

Articles

Behm FG, Raimondi SC, Frestedt JL, et al. Rearrangement of the MLL gene confers a poor prognosis in childhood acute lymphoblastic leukemia, regardless of presenting age. Blood 1996;87:2870–2877.

Borowitz MJ. Immunological markers in childhood acute lymphoblastic leukemia. Hematol Oncol Clin North Am 1990;4:743–765.

Borowitz MJ, Dowell BL, Boyett JM, et al. Monoclonal antibody definition of T cell acute leukemia: a Pediatric Oncology Group study. Blood 1985;65:785–788.

Chervinsky DS, Sait SN, Nowak NJ, et al. Complex MLL rearrangement in a patient with T-cell acute lymphoblastic leukemia. Genes Chromosom Cancer 1995;14:76–84.

Crist WM, Shuster JJ, Falletta J, et al. Clinical features and outcome in childhood T-cell leukemia-lymphoma according to stage of thymocyte differentiation: a Pediatric Oncology Group study. Blood 1988;72:1891–1897.

Kameko Y, Frizzera G, Shikano T, et al. Chromosomal and immunophenotypic patterns in T cell acute lymphoblastic leukemia (T ALL) and lymphoblastic lymphoma (LBL). Leukemia 1989;3:886–892.

Kobayashi H, Espinosa R III, Thirman MJ, et al. Heterogeneity of breakpoints of 11q23 rearrangements in hematologic malignancies identified with fluorescence in situ hybridization. Blood 1993;82:547–551.

LoCoco F, Mandelli F, Breccia M, et al. Southern blot analysis of ALL 1 rearrangements at chromosome 11q23 in acute leukemia. Cancer Res 1993;53:3800–3803.

McKenna RW, Parkin J, Brunning RD. Morphologic and ultrastructural characteristics of T-cell acute lymphoblastic leukemia. Cancer 1979;44:1290–1297.

Mirro J Jr, Kitchingman G, Behm FG, et al. T-cell differentiation stages identified by molecular and immunologic analysis of the T-cell receptor complex in childhood lymphoblastic leukemia. Blood 1987;69:908–912.

Raimondi SC, Frestedt JL, Pui CH, et al. Acute lymphoblastic leukemias with deletion of 11q23 or a novel inversion (11)(p13q23) lack MLL gene rearrangements and have favorable clinical features. Blood 1995;86:1881–1886.

Strout MP, Mrozek K, Heinonen K, et al. ML 1 cell line lacks a germline MLL locus. Genes Chromosom Cancer 1996;16:204–210.

Wodzinski MA, Watmore AE, Lilleyman JS, et al. Chromosomes in childhood acute lymphoblastic leukaemia: karyotypic patterns in disease subtypes. J Clin Pathol 1991;44:481–451.

Review Articles

Cortes JE, Kantarjian HM. Acute lymphoblastic leukemia. A comprehensive review with emphasis on biology and therapy. Cancer 1995;76:2393–2417.

CASE 9—BIPHENOTYPIC LEUKEMIA

B CELL/MYELOID LEUKEMIA

PATIENT: 14-year-old white female.

CHIEF COMPLAINT: Tiredness, fatigue, fever.

MEDICAL HISTORY: Patient was diagnosed in July 1990 with pre-B ALL CALLA+ and was treated with a standard risk protocol. Cytogenetics revealed a normal female karyotype. She relapsed 1 year later and was re-induced and received a bone marrow transplant in 1993. She relapsed in July 1996 with a hypodiploid karyotype, demonstrating three specific ALL changes, portending a poor prognosis. She was re-induced in the fall of 1996 and relapsed in April 1997. Despite additional treatment efforts she expired on April 29, 1997.

PHYSICAL EXAMINATION: Elevated temperature, no lymphadenopathy, hepatosplenomegaly.

CELL-DYN 4000® LABORATORY WORKSHEET

WBC (Viability)	3.92×10^9/L (55%)
Hemoglobin	10.8 g/dL
Platelets	27.2×10^9/L
Neutrophils	0.81×10^9/L (20.8%)
Monocytes	0.16×10^9/L (4%)
Eosinophils	0.02×10^9/L (0.6%)
Basophils	0.27×10^9/L (6.9%)
Lymphocytes	0.93×10^9/L (23.7%)
Variant Lymphs	1.68×10^9/L (43%)
Blasts	0.04×10^9/L (1.1%)
Suspect Flags	Blasts
	Variant Lymphs

The differential was difficult in this case, as in Case 8. Many atypical and bizarre lymphoid appearing cells were observed. The manual differential revealed 41% lymphocytes, 16% atypical lymphocytes, 16% blasts, 3% monocytes, 20% neutrophils, 3% bands, and 1% basophils (Fig. 8.18). As in the previous case, the analyzer had difficulty in sorting out the spectrum of lymphoid cells, but correctly flagged blasts, and variant lymphocytes. The number of viable cells (55%) was greatly reduced since the specimen was over 24 hours old (Fig. 8.19). This may be partially a pathological increase in permeability since normal peripheral blood cells do not show such loss in viability. d'Onofrio et al. showed that the nonviable WBC after 24 hours storage at 25°C was approximately 25%.

ADDITIONAL DATA: The bone marrow was very cellular and contained

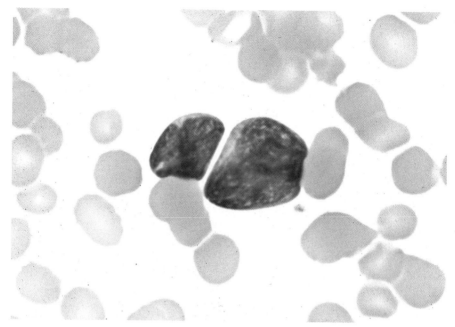

Figure 8.18. Peripheral blood showing atypical lymphoid cells and blasts (× 1000).

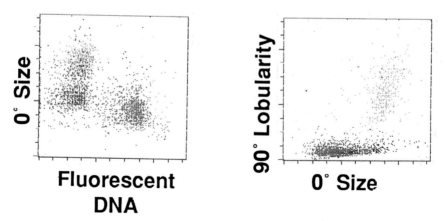

Figure 8.19. Scattergram (left) shows large number of non-viable lymphoid cells (blue) on right. Scattergram (right) shows expansion of lymphoid population (blue) indicating the presence of blasts and variant lymphocytes (purple).

large numbers of blasts with irregular, clefted nuclei. Many of the blasts contained prominent nucleoli.

Cytochemistry on the bone marrow revealed PAS+ granules within the lymphoid cells, MPEX−, SBB−, B-EST−, TdT+.

Flow cytometric analysis on the bone marrow revealed the abnormal lymphoid cells to be CD19+, CD13+, CD33+, HLA-DR+, and TdT+. Dual flow cytometric analysis showed CD19 and CD13, CD19 and CD33 positivity on the same cell population. The cells were cCD22+ and cCD3−.

Cytogenetics in July 1996 revealed a hypodiploid karyotype (n = 44) with ALL specific changes t(9p);t(12p);I(17q). Such changes would be expected to portend a very poor prognosis.

COMMENT: Confusion in terminology exists regarding classification of cases ranging from expression of one "aberrant" marker in otherwise typical ALL or AML to the more extreme instances of acute bilineage leukemia. The most useful discrimination is between bilineage and biphenotypic acute leukemia. The former indicates an acute leukemia with two separate blast populations, i.e., myeloid and lymphoid. The latter indicates cases where co-expression of lymphoid and myeloid markers occurs on the same cells. This was demonstrated in the current case. Various criteria have been utilized to define biphenotypic leukemia. Some authors classify cases as biphenotypic if two or more inappropriate markers are expressed; others have proposed more comprehensive schemes using morphologic, cytochemical, immunologic, and cytogenetic features. Catovsky et al. have relied mostly on immunophenotypic findings. Although the current patient was originally diagnosed as pre B-ALL CALLA+ with a normal karyotype, she progressed to a biphenotypic leukemia with multiple karyotypic abnormalities that predicted a poor outcome.

The left scattergram (Fig. 8.19) showed an increase in nonviable cells, possibly due to pathological increase in permeability and delay in analysis noted on the left. The nonviable cells are noted on the right side of the scattergram (blue). d'Onofrio et al. have shown that the percentage of leukocytes (ALL, CLL) permeable to propidium iodide was increased at baseline and even greater after 24 and 48 hours. The lymphoid population is expanded in both directions on the right scattergram. Also, purple dots to the right of the lymphoid population most likely represent blast cells.

BIBLIOGRAPHY

Articles

Buccheri V, Matutes E, Dyer MJ, et al. Lineage commitment in biphenotypic acute leukemia. Leukemia 1993;7:919–927.

d'Onofrio G, Zini G, Tommasi M, et al. Integration of fluorescence and hemocytometry in the Cell-Dyn 4000®: reticulocyte, nucleated red blood cell, and white blood cell viability study. Lab Hematol 1996;2:131–138.

Launder TM, Bray RA, Stempora L, et al. Lymphoid-associated antigen expression by acute myeloid leukemia. Am J Clin Pathol 1996;106:185–191.

Matutes E, Catovsky D. The value of scoring systems for the diagnosis of biphenotypic leukemia and mature KB-cell disorders. Leuk Lymphoma 1994;13:11–14.

Mirro J, Kitchingman CR. The morphology, cytochemistry, molecular characteristics, and clinical significance of acute mixed-lineage leukemia. In: Scott CS, ed. Leukemia cytochemistry: principles and practice. Chichester: Ellis Horwood, 1989.

Shetty V, Chitale A, Matutes E, et al. Immunological and ultrastructural studies in acute biphenotypic leukaemia. J Clin Path 1993;46:903–907.

Wood M, Palmer JH, Wright F, et al. Evaluation of complex chromosomal rearrangements in a case of biphenotypic pre-B/myeloid acute leukemia. Cancer Genet Cytogenet 1993;69:129–131.

Review Articles

Catovsky D, Matutes E. The classification of acute leukemia. Leukemia 1992;6(2):1–6.

Catovsky D, Matutes E, Buccheri V, et al. A classification of acute leukemia for the 1990s. Ann Hematol 1991;62:16–21.

Wang JC, Beauregard P, Soamboonsrup P, et al. Monoclonal antibodies in the management of acute leukemia. Am J Hematol 1995;50:188–199.

CASE 10—ACUTE MYELOID LEUKEMIA

FAB M7—ACUTE MEGAKARYOCYTIC LEUKEMIA

PATIENT: 77-year-old white female.

CHIEF COMPLAINT: Weakness, chronic fatigue, nausea

MEDICAL HISTORY: Patient was diagnosed with myeloid metaplasia with myelofibrosis in 1987. In the last year, she has become transfusion dependent. Bone marrow in March 1996 revealed greater than 90% fibrosis with marked reduction in normal marrow. Increased numbers of blast cells have appeared in the peripheral blood.

PHYSICAL EXAMINATION: Marked splenomegaly.

CELL-DYN 4000® LABORATORY WORKSHEET

WBC (Viability)	11.5×10^9/L (99%)
Hemoglobin	8.7 g/dL
Platelets	99.6×10^9/L
Neutrophils	3.7×10^9/L (32.3%)
Bands	0.23×10^9/L (2.04%)
Monocytes	0.28×10^9/L (2.48%)
Eosinophils	0.11×10^9/L (0.9%)
Lymphocytes	5.6×10^9/L (49%)
Variant Lymphs	0.024×10^9/L (0.2%)
IG	1.43×10^9/L (12.5%)
Blasts	0.08×10^9/L (0.7%)
NRBC	0.566×10^9 (4.48 NR/W)
Suspect Flags	IG
	Bands
	Blasts
	Variant Lymphs

The analyzer revealed increased lymphocytes, variant lymphs, bands, immature granulocytes, and blasts. It also detected nucleated red blood cells. The manual differential showed 12% lymphocytes, 31% blasts, 4% monocytes, 18% neutrophils, 15% bands, 10% metamyelocytes, 5% myelocytes, 5% promyelocytes, and 6% nucleated red blood cells. The instrument classified many of the blasts as lymphocytes; however, this is understandable since many of the blasts were micromegakaryoblasts (Fig. 8.20). The scattergram (Fig. 8.21) clearly showed expansion of the lymphocyte population (blue) and extension of the purple population to the right representing blasts (right scattergram).

ADDITIONAL DATA: Bone marrow aspirate was unobtainable. The bone marrow biopsy showed marked fibrosis with scattered nests of blasts.

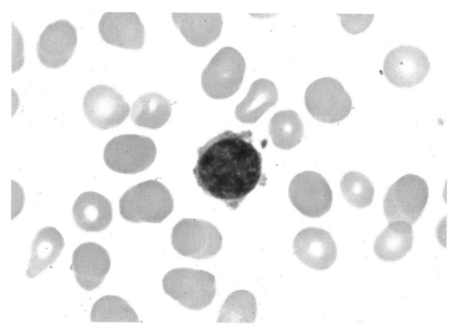

Figure 8.20. Peripheral blood showing micromegakaryoblast. Note budding platelets (× 1000).

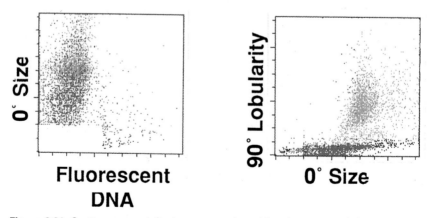

Figure 8.21. Scattergram on left shows expansion of lymphocyte population (blue). Scattergram on right shows expansion of lymphocyte population and presence of blasts (purple, far right).

Cytochemistry and TdT on the peripheral blood blasts: MPEX−, SBB−, A-EST+, fluoride sensitive, B-EST−, PAS+ localized granular pattern, and TdT−. Immunoalkaline phosphatase on peripheral blood blasts CD41+, CD42b+.

Flow cytometric analysis on the peripheral blood revealed CD13+, CD33+, CD41+, CD426+, CD61+, and CD36+.

Immunohistochemistry on the bone marrow biopsy revealed nests of blasts to be Factor VIII+. Electron microscopy for platelet peroxidase was positive. Cytogenetics were not performed.

COMMENT: The incidence of acute megakaryocytic leukemia FAB M7 is 8 to 10% of AML cases. The cells are highly pleomorphic; ranging from small round cells with scant amounts of cytoplasm and dense, heavy chromatin, sometimes resembling lymphoblasts (L1), to cells that more closely resemble the L2 lymphoblasts with or without granules, with one to three nucleoli. As in this case, the cells may demonstrate cytoplasmic blebs, and platelets may be observed extending from the surface. Since the bone marrow is fibrotic in cases of myeloid metaplasia with myelofibrosis, some authors have implied that leukemic transformation arises in the peripheral blood. Also, blast transformation could occur in extramedullary sites such as lymph nodes, liver, or spleen; however, the lung may be the likely source of megakaryoblasts because it has long been known that megakaryocytes reside in this organ. Therefore, the lungs deserve scrutiny as a source for the possible origin of megakaryoblasts in this unique form of acute leukemia.

The scattergram showed a marked expansion of the lymphocyte area (blue) in both scattergrams. This was related to the lymphoid morphology of the circulating blasts. Note the extension of the blasts (purple) to the right in lobularity/size scattergram.

BIBLIOGRAPHY

Articles

Akahoshi M, Oshimi K, Mizoguchi H, et al. Myeloproliferative disorders terminating in acute megakaryoblastic leukemia with chromosome 3q26 abnormality. Cancer 1987;60:2654–2661.

Breton-Gorius J, Vanhaeke D, Pryzwansky KB, et al. Simultaneous detection of membrane markers with monoclonal antibodies and peroxidatic activities in leukemia: ultrastructural analysis using a new method of fixation preserving the platelet peroxidase. Br J Haematol 1984;58:447–458.

Efrati P, Nir E, Yaari A, et al. Myeloproliferative disorders terminating in acute micromegakaryoblastic leukemia. Br J Haematol 1980;43:79–86.

Fisher D, Ruchlemer R, Hiller N, et al. Aggressive bone destruction in acute megakaryocytic leukemia: a rare presentation. Pediatr Radiol 1997;27:20–22.

Huang M, Li C-Y, Nichols WL, et al. Acute leukemia with megakaryocytic differentiation: a study of 12 cases identified immunocytochemically. Blood 1984;64:427–439.

Marcus RE, Hibbin JA, Matutes E, et al. Megakaryoblastic transformation of myelofibrosis with expression of the c-sis oncogene. Scand J Haematol 1986;36:186–193.

Review Articles

Bennett JM, Catovsky D, Daniel MT, et al. Criteria for the diagnosis of acute leukemias of megakaryocytic lineage (M7). Ann Int Med 1985;103:406–462.
Breton-Gorius J. Review of the ultra-structure and cytochemistry of megakaryoblastic leukemia. In: Polliak A. Human leukemias. Boston: Martinus Nijhoff, 1984:63–92.
Gassmann W, Loffler H. Acute megakaryoblastic leukemia. Leukemia Lymphoma 1995;1:69–73.
Patino-Sarcinelli F, Knecht H, Pechet L, et al. Leukemia with megakaryocytic differentiation following essential thrombocythemia and myelofibrosis. Case report and review of the literature. Acta Haematologica 1996;95:122–128.
Yamaguchi K, Shimamura K. Pulmonary fibrosis with megakaryocytoid cell infiltration and chronic myelogenous leukemia. Leukemia Lymphoma 1994;15:253–259.

CHAPTER 9

Bone Marrow Evaluation by Cell-Dyn 4000® System

GENERAL COMMENTS

This portion of the book represents a new way of evaluating bone marrows by automated hematologic instrumentation. The Cell-Dyn 4000® system employs optical and fluorescent technology that makes it feasible to analyze bone marrow cells. Although the instrument is not FDA 510(k) cleared for this application, current research will help in the automation of bone marrow screening. In our experience in evaluating over 100 bone marrows, we have found that those marrows placed directly into heparin give comparable results to those collected in heparin and RPMI medium and processed for flow cytometric analysis.

This would eliminate filtering through a stainless steel mesh, nylon mesh, and washing in phosphate buffered saline; however, if heparin marrow is evaluated by the Cell-Dyn 4000® system, care should be taken to make sure the specimen is well mixed and does not contain large marrow particles or clots. This section focuses on the acute leukemias, but marrows with variable hematological disorders can be appraised by automated analysis. This could be used to give initial information prior to the bone marrow sign out similar to the current use of basic hematological information generated on the peripheral blood. Most physicians in our institution do not evaluate scattergrams on the peripheral blood of their patients. Nevertheless, our technologists responsible for reporting complete blood counts (CBCs) constantly rely on these screens.

The reader should take note as to how the Cell-Dyn 4000® system's automated technology classifies blast cells. With our limited experience, we can already see patterns emerging that give important diagnostic information. Especially note the AML M4Eo patient before and after treatment. The blast cells and abnormal eosinophils were eliminated by chemotherapy. This was confirmed by examination of the bone marrow aspirate, biopsy, and clot. Also, note the blast cells are separated by size, nuclear shape, and presence of granules (type II blasts). Furthermore, the Cell-Dyn 4000® system has an Argon laser that gives it the capability to analyze fluorescent monoclonal antibodies used in flow cytometers. This will give the added future advantage of performing a complete hematological analysis by utilizing one instrument rather than two. In these days of cost containment, reduction in personnel, and improved efficiency such an instrument should have great appeal in the marketplace of the future.

225

The future is upon us! If a chess computer (Deep Blue) can trounce the world international grand master, then, within the foreseeable future, automated instrumentation should be able to interpret peripheral bloods and bone marrows as well, or better than, hematologists and hematopathologists. Does this mean we are all out of a job? Nonsense! The hematologists and hematopathologists of the future will graduate to more sophisticated levels of analysis involving cytokines, molecular genetics, and discoveries as yet unknown. Nevertheless, there will be many of us in the near future, by nature of our training, peering down a microscope looking at the beautiful array of cells in peripheral blood and bone marrow establishing diagnoses.

BONE MARROW CASE 1

NONDIAGNOSTIC BONE MARROW

The experimental data on this nondiagnostic bone marrow are listed in Table 9.1. Note that the left column represents the absolute numbers, and the right column represents the percentages. Immature granulocytes (IG) account for 7.9% of the marrow population and blasts account for 1.97%. The Cell-Dyn 4000® M:E ratio is calculated from [WBC − (LYMe + VARL)/NRBC]. The instrument's calculated M:E was 4.5:1 compared to an estimated 4:1.

The size versus FL3 (DNA fluorescence) scatterplot on the left (Fig. 9.1A) show large nonfluorescent viable leukocytes. Similar sized nonviable leukocytes with increased fluorescence appear above the small fluorescent NRBC (red). Note that leukocyte viability of the sample is 90.3% (Table 9.1). The NRBC (red) are composed of two populations. The least fluorescent population is probably the least mature. The more fluorescent population is probably the most mature. The lobularity versus size scatterplot on the right (Fig. 9.1A) shows a heterogeneous neutrophil population (orange) with events in the immature granulocyte region to the right and nonviable neutrophils to the left of the major population. Bands decrease lobularity and lower the center of the neutrophil population. Blasts increase the heterogeneity of the monocyte population (purple). Some of the dots (purple) to the far right most likely represent blasts. A photomicrograph of this nondiagnostic marrow is depicted in Fig. 9.1B.

Table 9.1
Nondiagnostic Bone Marrow Hemogram from Cell–Dyn Laboratory Worksheet

WBC	15.1*10e3/µL	WVF	.903*
SEG	8.88*	%S	58.9*
BAND	2.54*	%BD	16.8*
IG	1.19*	%IG	7.90*
BLST	.297*	%BL	1.97*
MONe	.134*	%Me	.886*
EOS	.330*	%E	2.19*
BASO	.065*	%B	.429*
LYMe	1.65*	%Le	10.9*
VARL	0.00*	%VL	0.00*
NRBC	3.00*10e3/µL	NR/W 19.9*	

Some events rules "out of bounds."

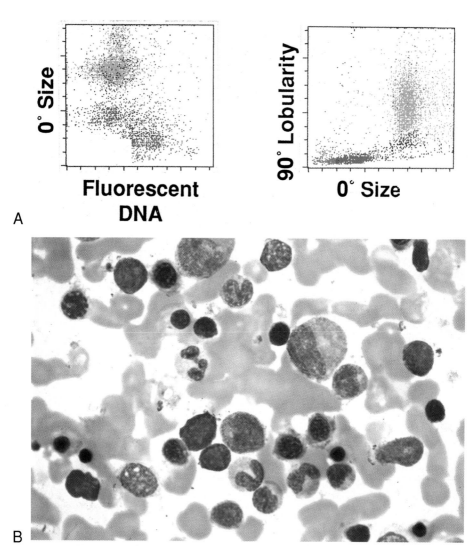

Figure 9.1. A. Scatterplots of a nondiagnostic bone marrow evaluated by the cell-dyn 4000®. Scatterplot on the left shows size versus FL3 (fluorescent DNA). This separates the marrow cells into granulocytic (orange), eosinophilic (green), monocytic (purple), lymphocytic (blue) and nucleated red blood cells (NRBC-red). In addition, it determines cell viability. Scatterplot on the right shows lobularity versus size. This separates the cells in such a way that blast cells may be easily detected. B. Microphotograph of nondiagnostic bone marrow (× 400).

BIBLIOGRAPHY

Articles

Islam A. Hemopoietic stem cell: a new concept. Leukemia Res 1985;9:1415–1432.

Loken MR, Shah VO, Dattilio KL, et al. Flow cytometric analysis of human bone marrow: II. Normal B lymphocyte development. Blood 1987;70:1316–1324.

Ogawa M. Differentiation and proliferation of hematopoietic stem cells. Blood 1993;81:2844–2853.

Review Articles

Burkhardt R. Bone marrow in megakaryocytic disorders. Hematol Oncol Clin North Am 1988;4:695–733.

Foucar K. Bone marrow pathology. Chicago: American Society of Clinical Pathologists Press, 1995.

Gewirtz AM. Human megakaryocytopoiesis. Semin Hematol 1986;23:27–42.

Gulati GL, Ashton JK, Hyun BH. Structure and function of the bone marrow and hematopoiesis. Hematol Oncol Clin North Am 1988;2:495–511.

Krantz SB. Erythropoietin. Blood 1991;77:419–434.

Larson RS, McCurley TL. Cutting edge technologies in the evaluation of bone marrow samples. Clin Lab Sci 1996;9(6):354–357.

Nathan DG. Regulation of hematopoiesis. Pediatr Res 1990;27:423–431.

Wickramasinghe SN. Bone marrow. In: Sternberg SS, ed. Histology for pathologists. New York: Raven Press, 1992:1–31.

Williams WJ. Hematology. 5th ed. New York: McGraw-Hill, 1995:15–38.

BONE MARROW CASE 2

ACUTE MYELOMONOCYTIC LEUKEMIA
WITH EOSINOPHILIA AML M4Eo

The experimental data on the bone marrow from this patient are shown in Table 9.2. Note the marked increase in blasts (23.1%) and eosinophils (26.3%). This is in striking contrast to the hemogram on the nondiagnostic bone marrow. The size versus FL3 (DNA fluorescence) scatterplot (left) (Fig. 9.2A) shows expansion into the granulocytic area (orange) creating a dark (purple to black) spot. This most likely represents the blasts and immature leukemic elements. The eosinophils are also in this region. The lobularity versus the size scatterplot (right) (Fig. 9.2A) reveals the eosinophils (green) and the blasts (purple). A photomicrograph of the bone marrow demonstrating the blast cells and eosinophils with basophilic granules is shown (Fig. 9.2B).

After 2 weeks of treatment, the patient was re-evaluated by bone marrow examination. The experimental data are shown in Table 9.3. Note that the blasts are 0% and the eosinophils markedly diminished from the onset marrow. The scattergrams are shown in Figure 9.2C. Note the blasts have disappeared and eosinophils have markedly decreased. The microphotograph (Fig. 9.2D) shows normal bone marrow.

Table 9.2
Acute Myelomonocytic Leukemia With Eosinophilia (AML M4Eo) Hemogram from Cell–Dyn 4000 Laboratory Worksheet Before Therapy

WBC	14.8*10e3/μL	WVF	.906*
SEG	2.41*	%S	16.3*
BAND	1.34*	%BD	9.06*
IG	1.02*	%IG	6.87*
BLST	3.43*	%BL	23.1*
MONe	1.18*	%Me	8.00*
EOS	3.90*	%E	26.3*
BASO	.051*	%B	.348*
LYMe	1.47*	%Le	9.96*
VARL	0.00*	%VL	0.00*
NRBC	1.55*10e3/μL	NR/W 10.5*	

*Some events rules "out of bounds."

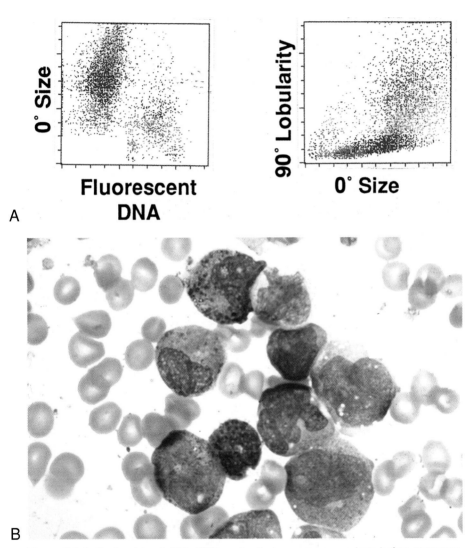

Figure 9.2 A. Scatterplots of AML M4Eo patient's bone marrow aspirate before treatment. Note events in blast region (purple) and abnormal eosinophils. B. Bone marrow aspirate with blasts and abnormal eosinophils (AML M4Eo) before therapy (× 1000). C. Scatterplots of AML M4Eo patient's bone marrow aspirate after therapy. Note absence of events in blast region, and decline in eosinophils. Note remaining eosinophils have shifted position probably due to fact they are normal. D. Normal appearance of bone marrow aspirate after treatment (× 400).

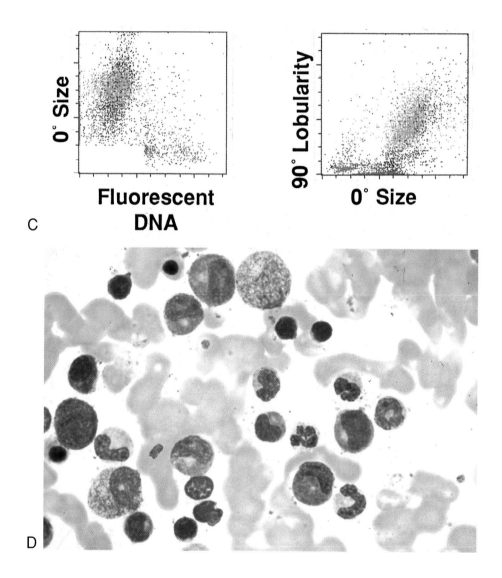

C

D

Table 9.3
Acute Myelomonocytic Leukemia With Eosinophilia (AML M4Eo) Hemogram from Cell–Dyn Laboratory Worksheet After Therapy

WBC	17.1*10e3/μL	WVF	.951*
SEG	9.53*	%S	55.9*
BAND	0.00*	%BD	0.00*
IG	.910*	%IG	5.34*
BLST	0.00*	%BL	0.00*
MONe	.220*	%Me	1.29*
EOS	1.50*	%E	8.81*
BASO	.363*	%B	2.13*
LYMe	4.53*	%Le	26.6*
VARL	0.00*	%VL	0.00*
NRBC	1.40*10e3/μL	NR/W	8.20*

Some events rules "out of bounds."

BIBLIOGRAPHY

Articles

Berger R, Derre J, LeConiat M, et al. Inversion-associated translocations in acute myelomonocytic leukemia with eosinophilia. Genes Chromosom Cancer 1995;12(1):58–62.

Haferlach T, Gasmann W, Loffler H, et al. Clinical aspects of acute myeloid leukemias of the FAB types M3 and M4Eo. The AML Cooperative Group. Ann Hematol 1993;66(4):165–170.

Monohan BP, Rector JT, Liu PP, et al. Clinical aspects of expression of inversion 16 chromosomal fusion transcript CBFB/MYH11 in acute myelogenous leukemia subtype M1 with abnormal bone marrow eosinophilia. Leukemia 1996;10:1653–1654.

Review Articles

Brunning RD, McKenna RW. Acute leukemias. In: Brunning RD, McKenna RW. Atlas of tumor pathology: tumors of the bone marrow. Fascicle 9. Washington, DC: AFILP, 1994:53–56.

Foucar K. Bone marrow pathology. Chicago: American Society of Clinical Pathologists Press, 1995.

Haferlach T, Winkemann M, Loffler H, et al. The abnormal eosinophils are part of the leukemic cell population in acute myelomonocytic leukemia with abnormal eosinophils (AML M4Eo) and carry the pericentric inversion 16: a combination of May-Grunwald-Giemsa staining and fluorescence in situ hybridization. Blood 1996; 87(6):2459–2463.

Liu PP, Hajra A, Wijmenga C, et al. Molecular pathogenesis of the chromosome 16 inversion in the M4Eo subtype of acute myeloid leukemia. Blood 1995; 85(9):2289–2302.

Schumacher HR. Acute leukemia. Approach to diagnosis. New York: Igaku-Shoin, 1990.

BONE MARROW CASE 3

ACUTE MYELOMONOCYTIC LEUKEMIA AML M4

The experimental data on this case are shown in Table 9.4. Note that the blast population constitutes 33.6% of the bone marrow cells. Also, the eosinophils only constituted 5.45% of the bone marrow cells. The size versus FL3 (DNA fluorescence) scatterplot (left) (Fig. 9.3A) shows expansion into the granulocytic area (orange) creating a large black-purple spot. These most likely represent blasts and immature granulocytic-monocytic precursors. The lobularity versus the size scatterplot (right) (Fig. 9.3A) shows an increase in events in the blast (purple) and immature granulocyte region (orange). The purple/orange intersection forms a line bisecting the abnormal populations (monocytic, granulocytic). A photomicrograph of the bone marrow is demonstrated (Fig. 9.3B). Observe the large numbers of blast cells.

Table 9.4
Acute Myelomonocytic Leukemia AML M4 Hemogram
from Cell–Dyn 4000® Laboratory Worksheet

WBC	12.5*10e3/µL	WVF	.806*
SEG	2.54*	%S	20.4*
BAND	.282*	%BD	2.27*
IG	.063*	%IG	.503*
BLST	4.19*	%BL	33.6*
MONe	2.07*	%Me	16.6*
EOS	.680*	%E	5.45*
BASO	.088*	%B	.705*
LYMe	1.62*	%Le	13.0*
VARL	.933*	%VL	7.48*
NRBC	.897*10e3/µL	NR/W	7.20*

Some events ruled "out of bounds."

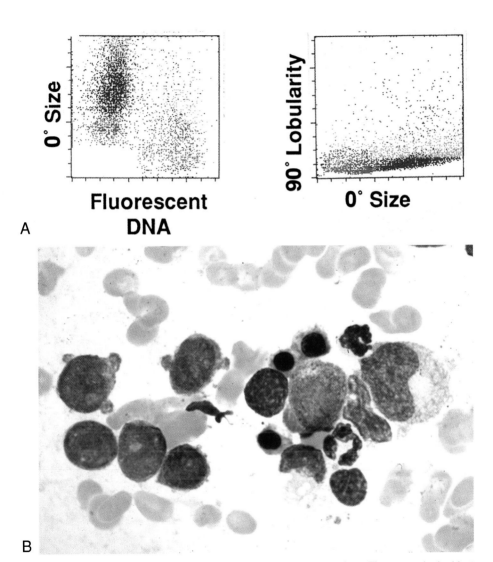

Figure 9.3. A. Scatterplots of AML M4 patient's bone marrow aspirate. The events in the blast and immature regions are purple, and orange. The lobularity versus size scatterplot demonstrates a line between the abnormal granulocytic (orange) and monocytic elements (purple). B. Microphotograph showing bone marrow (✕ 400).

BIBLIOGRAPHY

Articles

Bower ML, Parry P, Carter M, et al. Prevalence and clinical correlations of MLL gene rearrangements in AML M4/5. Blood 1994;84(11):3776–3780.

Bruno A, Del Poeta G, Venditti A, et al. Diagnosis of acute myeloid leukemia and system Coulter VCS. Haematologica 1994;79(5):420–428.

Cimino G, Rapanotti MC, Elia L, et al. ALL-1 gene rearrangements in acute myeloid leukemia: association with M4-M5 French-American-British classification subtypes and young age. Cancer Res 1995;15:1625–1628.

Hoo JJ, Gregory SA, Jones B, et al. Supernumerary isochromosome 4p in ANLL M4 myelomonocytic type is associated with favorable prognosis. Cancer Genet Cytogenet 1995;79(2):127–129.

Jansen JH, Fibbe WE, Wientjens GJ, et al. Inhibitory effect of interleukin-4 on the proliferation of acute myeloid leukemia cells with myelo-monocytic differentiation (AML M4/M5); the role of interleukin-6. Leukemia 1993;7(4):643–645.

Koyama A, Shsirakawa C, Masaki H, et al. Factors related to prognosis and relapse in acute myelomonocytic and monocytic leukemias (M4 and M5). Rinsho Ketsueki 1990;31(11):1787–1793.

Terstappen LW, Konemann S, Safford M, et al. Flow cytometric characterization of acute myeloid leukemia. Part 1. Significance of light scattering properties. Leukemia 1991;5(4):315–321.

Review Articles

Brunning RD, McKenna RW. Acute leukemias: In: Brunning RD, McKenna RW. Atlas of tumor pathology: tumors of the bone marrow. Fascicle 9. Washington, DC: AFIP, 1994:53–56.

Foucar K. Bone marrow pathology. Chicago: American Society of Clinical Pathologists Press, 1995.

Schumacher HR. Acute leukemia. Approach to diagnosis. New York: Igaku-Shoin, 1990.

BONE MARROW CASE 4

ACUTE MYELOGENOUS LEUKEMIA AML M1

The experimental data from the patient's bone marrow aspirate are shown in Table 9.5. Note that the blasts are elevated. Interestingly, these blasts were characterized as lymphocytes with increased heterogeneity. The extreme heterogeneity in this single population resulted in the instrument classifying the larger cells as variant lymphocytic and the very largest cells as blasts. This situation could easily be resolved in the instrument with a few appropriately selected monoclonal antibodies such as myeloperoxidase, CD 13,

Table 9.5
Acute Myelogenous Leukemia Without Maturation AML M1 Hemogram from Cell–Dyn 4000® Laboratory Worksheet

WBC	4.47 10e3/µL	WVF	.964
SEG	.195	%S	4.37
BAND	.002	%BD	.042
IG	.008	%IG	.170
BLST	.085*	%BL	1.91*
MONe	.019*	%Me	.424*
EOS	.019	%E	.424
BASO	.004	%B	.085
LYMe	4.02*	%Le	89.9*
VARL	.120*	%VL	2.67*
NRBC	0.0010e3/µL	NR/W	0.00

Some events ruled "out of bounds."

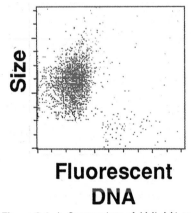
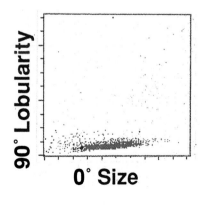

Figure 9.4. A. Scatterplots of AML M1 patient's bone marrow aspirate. The expanded lymphocyte area in the scatterplots in the increased size areas represent the blast cells. B. Microphotograph showing the blast cells. Note high N/C ratio and lymphoid appearance of these small micromyeloblasts (× 400).

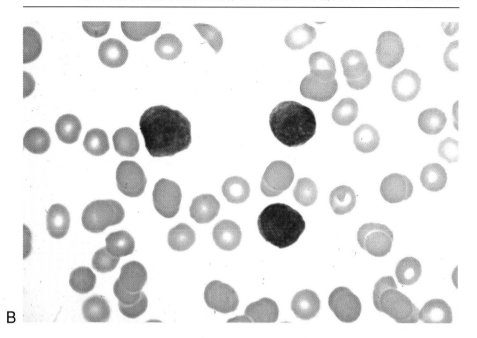

B

CD 33 (Fig. 9.4A). The photomicrograph (Fig. 9.4B) shows small blasts with a high N/C ratio and lymphoid appearance. From cytochemical and flow analysis these were found to be micromyeloblasts.

BIBLIOGRAPHY

Articles

Bruno A, Del Poeta G, Venditti A, et al. Diagnosis of acute myeloid leukemia and system Coulter VCS. Haematologica 1994;79:420–428.

Del Poeta G, Stasi R, Venditti A, et al. Prognostic value of cell marker analysis in de novo acute myeloid leukemia. Leukemia 1994;8:388–394.

Hamamoto K, Date M, Taniguchi H, et al. Heterogeneity of acute myeloblastic leukemia without maturation: an ultrastructural study. Ultrastruct Pathol 1995; 19(1): 9–14.

Poirel H, Rack K, Delabesse E, et al. Incidence and characterization of MLL gene (11q23) rearrangements in acute myeloid leukemia M1 and M5. Blood 1996; 87:2496–2505.

Wells SJ, Bray RA, Stempora LL, et al. CD117/CD34 expression in leukemic blasts. Am J Clin Pathol 1996;106:192–195.

Review Articles

Brunning RD, McKenna RW. Acute leukemias. In: Brunning RD, McKenna RW. Atlas of tumor pathology: tumors of the bone marrow. Fascicle 9. Washington, DC: AFIP, 1994;32–37.

Foucar K. Bone marrow pathology. Chicago: American Society of Clinical Pathologists Press, 1995.

Rohatiner A, Lister TA. Acute myelogenous leukemia in adults. In: Henderson ES, Lister TA, Greaves MF. Leukemia. 6th ed. Philadelphia: WB Saunders, 1996:479–512.

Schumacher HR. Acute leukemia: approach to diagnosis. New York: Igaku-Shoin, 1990.

BONE MARROW CASE 5

ACUTE ERYTHROLEUKEMIA, AML M6A

The experimental data on this case are listed in Table 9.6. The erythroid precursors appear as lymphocytes, variant lymphocytes, and NRBC. The M:E ratio calculated by the original formula was 0.6:1. Adding lymphocytes and variant lymphocytes to the NRBC, as well as subtracting them from the WBC, resulted in a more accurate M:E ratio 0.3:1 (manual 0.23:1). More of the cells may have been correctly identified as NRBC by extended lysis and staining time in the resistant RBC mode. The scatterplots demonstrate the marked extension into the lymphocyte (blue) area by the abnormal red cell

Table 9.6
Acute Erythroleukemia M6a Hemogram
from Cell–Dyn 4000® Laboratory Worksheet

WBC	8.40*10e3/µL	WVF	.741
SEG	1.64*	%S	19.5*
BAND	.576*	%BD	6.86*
IG	.159*	%IG	1.90*
BLST	.372*	%BL	4.42*
MONe	.408*	%Me	4.86*
EOS	.118*	%E	1.41*
BASO	.031*	%B	.365*
LYMe	3.49*	%Le	41.6*
VARL	1.61*	%VL	19.1*
NRBC	5.89*10e3/µL	NR/W	70.1*

Some events ruled "out of bounds."

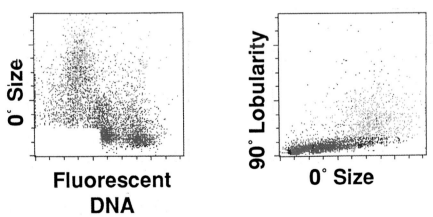

Fluorescent DNA

0° Size

A

Figure 9.5. A. Scatterplots of AML M6a patient's bone marrow aspirate with erythroid elements extending into lymphocyte area. B. Bone marrow showing numerous erythroid precursors with some scattered myeloblasts (× 400).

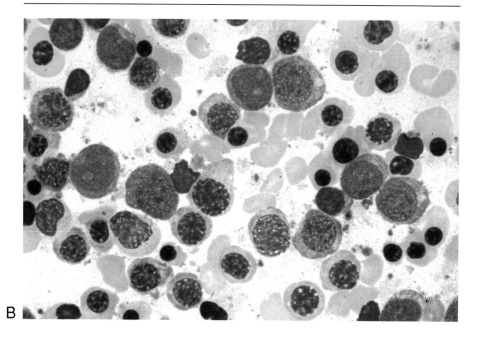

B

precursors (red) (Fig. 9.5A). The bone marrow aspirate (Fig. 9.5B) shows large numbers of erythroid precursors. Note the presence of myeloblasts with nucleoli and moderate amounts of blue-gray cytoplasm.

BIBLIOGRAPHY

Articles

Cuneo A, Van Orshoven A, Michaux JL, et al. Morphologic, immunologic, and cytogenetic studies in erythroleukemia: evidence for multilineage involvement and identification of two distinct cytogenetic-clinicopathological types. Br J Haematol 1990;75:346–354.

Davey FR, Abraham N Jr, Brunetto VL, et al. Morphologic characteristics of erythroleukemia (acute myeloid leukemia; FAB M6): a CALGB study. Am J Hematol 1995;49(1):29–38.

Kowal-Vern A, Cotelingam JD, Schumacher HR. The prognostic significance of proerythroblasts in acute erythroleukemia. Am J Clin Pathol 1992;98(1):34–40.

Laskin WB, Cotelingam JD, Duval-Arnould B, et al. Erythroleukemia in a child: value of immunocytochemistry and transmission electron microscopy in its diagnosis. Am J Pediatr Hematol Oncol 1985;7:99–103.

Olopade OI, Thangavelu M, Larson RA, et al. Clinical, morphologic, and cytogenetic characteristics of 26 patients with acute erythroblastic leukemia. Blood 1992;80:2873–2882.

Siebert R, Jhanwar S, Brown K, et al. Familial acute myeloid leukemia and Di Guglielmo syndrome. Leukemia 1995;9(6):1091–1094.

Review Articles

Brunning RD, McKenna RW. Acute leukemias. In: Brunning RD, McKenna RW. Atlas of tumor pathology: tumors of the bone marrow. Fascicle 9. Washington, DC: AFIP, 1994:67–77.

Foucar K. Bone marrow pathology. Chicago: American Society of Clinical Pathologists Press, 1995.

Grignani F, Testa U, Fagioli M, et al. Oncogenes and erythroid differentiation. Semin Can Biol 1994;5:125–135.

Schumacher HR. Acute leukemia: approach to diagnosis. New York: Igaku-Shoin, 1990.

Index

References in *italics* denote figures; those followed by "t" denote tables